Type A Behavior: Its Diagnosis and Treatment

PREVENTION IN PRACTICE LIBRARY

SERIES EDITOR
Thomas P. Gullotta
Child and Family Agency, New London, Connecticut

TYPE A BEHAVIOR: ITS DIAGNOSIS AND TREATMENT
Meyer Friedman

Type A Behavior: Its Diagnosis and Treatment

Meyer Friedman

Meyer Friedman Institute
Mount Zion Medical Center
University of California, San Francisco
San Francisco, California

Plenum Press • New York and London

Library of Congress Cataloging-in-Publication Data

On file

ISBN 0-306-45356-8 (Hardbound)
ISBN 0-306-45357-6 (Paperback)

© 1996 Plenum Press, New York
A Division of Plenum Publishing Corporation
233 Spring Street, New York, N. Y. 10013

10 9 8 7 6 5 4 3 2 1

To William S. Breall,
my esteemed cardiologist and friend,
whose efforts founded the Meyer Friedman Institute

Preface to the Series

In 1976, the National Institute of Mental Health held a working conference with the title, "Primary Prevention: An Idea Whose Time Has Come." That same year, a group in Vermont began an occasional series of books and symposia devoted to promoting health and preventing physical and emotional illness. How bold and farsighted those individuals were. In 1976, the focus of North American healthcare was not on prevention. Far from it; healthcare concerns were focused on how medical technology could restore functioning in bodies wasted by years of oftentimes conscious emotional and physical neglect and mistreatment. Gradually, as the costs of this remarkable but individually focused medical technology began to threaten the economic health of North American nations, attention shifted from technological and pharmacological advances to cost-containment strategies. We are in the midst of that new emerging cost-conscious healthcare treatment paradigm. Within that paradigm, the concept of primary prevention has arrived. It has arrived because it is far better to prevent heart disease than to perform by-pass surgery. It is better to encourage bicycling, skating, and motorcycle helmets than to provide rehabilitation services to a traumatically brain-injured individual. When we can identify in early childhood those youth who will be in likely contact with the law, it is wiser and more humane to help these socially impaired young people develop needed social skills than to incarcerate them in adolescence.

This series of monographs is an outgrowth of the dramatic changes that are occurring in the delivery of healthcare. Practitioners, whether they be physicians, psychologists, social workers, nurses, marriage and family therapists, or educators, recognize that their current skills need to be widened to include preventive interventions. Fortunately, there is an existing, theoretically driven and empirically proven technology available to those who wish to incorporate prevention into their practice.

This monograph series will share with practitioners prevention's technology in a very practical and applied manner. What is prevention's technology? Prevention uses four tools to promote health and reduce the incidence of illness. The tools are: education, social competency enhancement, natural caregiving, and systems change. In each of the monographs that appear in this series, readers will see how two or more of these technologies can be brought together to effect change.

For example, in Dr. Meyer Friedman's monograph, *Type A Behavior: Its Diagnosis and Treatment*, the reader will see how he uses education and social support to alter very destructive behavioral patterns to improve coronary health and social behavior. I am very pleased to be able to introduce this series with an author whose scholarship and medical practice are respected throughout the world. In future monographs, other distinguished scholars and practitioners will be sharing their preventive techniques on important issues such as positive aging, healthy sexuality, attention-deficit disorder, alcohol and drug prevention, and curbing violence.

Finally, I share with my treatment colleagues the reality that primary prevention is not a panacea. It does not offer a utopia. It does not promise health to all. Nor does it promise health to some for all time. It will not replace the need for treatment. Rather, primary prevention is about putting into daily practice good health practices on an individual, family, and societal basis to reduce the overall incidence of physical and emotional ill health. When one considers the incidence of serious illness in North America and the real good for millions of people that would result from reducing that incidence by merely 10%, the wisdom of moving that knowledge into the hands of practitioners and the public makes sense.

Thomas P. Gullotta
Child and Family Agency
New London, Connecticut

Preface

In 1959, Dr. Ray H. Rosenman and I first pointed out that a strong relationship existed between coronary heart disease and what we described as type A behavior (TAB). It was not until 1979, however, that my colleagues and I began the Recurrent Coronary Prevention Project (RCPP). We attempted and succeeded in modifying the intensity of TAB exhibited in approximately 400 postinfarction patients. Such patients, over a period of 4.5 years, experienced 45% fewer cardiac recurrences than the control patients. Much of what we learned about how to diagnose and quantitatively assess the intensity of TAB was accomplished in this study, which incidentally was the first study ever done to successfully modify TAB in postinfarction patients.

I have tried, in writing this volume, to describe diagnostic and intervention procedures, which, if followed, should enable not only psychologists, psychiatrists, and internists but also individuals who have received their doctorate in education to moderate type A behavior. I say this because, of the 20 group leaders who presently are modifying TAB in our ongoing research project, several are educators and their success in altering the TAB pattern is as good as that achieved by the psychologists, psychiatrists, and internists now leading groups of TAB persons at the Friedman Institute. I should add that sociologists, too, on occasion, have learned how to become successful TAB interventionists.

I believe it is appropriate at this juncture to give credit to those colleagues of mine who played salient roles in the RCPP. They were William S. Breall, MD; Stephen Elek, MD; Nancy Fleischmann, BA; Richard Levy, MD; Virginia Price, PhD; David Rabin, MD; Carl Thoresen, PhD; and Diane Ulmer, MS.

I also wish to express my thanks to Paul Bracke, PhD, who was of great importance in planning the general thrust of this book. Finally, I am deeply indebted to my office assistant, Diane P. Remillard, who was indispensable in the preparation of the manuscript for this book.

Contents

I

General Understanding and Medical Diagnosis of Type A Behavior

1

Overview of Types A and B Behavior

We shall first describe the specific psychopathological characteristics that comprise this disorder and then describe the resultant neurological, hormonal, and metabolic dysfunctions observed in this syndrome. The possible pathological effects of the disorder on the structure of coronary plaques also will be discussed.

THE PSYCHOPATHOLOGICAL CHARACTERISTICS OF TYPE A BEHAVIOR

The characteristics consist of both covert and overt components. The covert and, I believe, the causative factor responsible for the initiation and continuance of type A behavior (TAB) is an intrinsic insecurity or an insufficient degree of self-esteem.

Although only a minority of psychologists and psychiatrists (Gatson & Teevan, 1980; Houston & Vavack, 1991; Price, Friedman, Fleischmann, & Ghandour, 1995), who have or are still investigating TAB, are aware of the covert component, almost all of them are cognizant of the overt emotional disturbances peculiar to this disorder.

The most commonly observed overt characteristic of TAB is the sense of time urgency or impatience that is felt and manifested by almost all TAB subjects (Friedman & Rosenman, 1959; Price, 1982; Review Panel on Coronary-Prone Behavior, 1981). Frequently, this impatience becomes so intense that it creates and sustains a chronic sense of irritation or exasperation.

3

The second overt emotional TAB manifestation is what we have designated free-floating hostility. Very early in our studies (Friedman & Rosenman, 1974), I employed the adjective "free-floating" in describing TAB hostility because of the ubiquity and triviality of the incidents that can evoke hostility. Both the covert and the two overt TAB components will be described in detail in subsequent chapters.

THE NEUROLOGICAL DYSFUNCTIONS OF TAB

There is almost no doubt that the sympathetic nervous system is hyperactive more or less chronically in subjects suffering from TAB. Long ago, Walter Cannon (1915), in his classic monograph, demonstrated that when one animal struggles against another, the sympathetic nervous system hyperreacts. Were Cannon alive today, I feel reasonably certain that he would recognize that when modern man struggles against time or other persons, the conflict, as far as nature perceives it, is identical with that of one animal struggling against another.

Just as Cannon observed in 1915 that the blood-clotting time of his fighting cats hastened, we observed 42 years later (Friedman, Rosenman & Carroll, 1958) that the blood-clotting time of accountants similarly hastened as they struggled not against each other but against time to complete all of their clients' tax returns before the April 15 deadline. Again, as Cannon observed that his struggling cats secreted excess epinephrine, so my associates and I (Friedman, St. George, Byers, & Rosenman, 1960) and Williams and his associates (Williams et al., 1982) observed later that TAB subjects who were struggling against time and other persons also secreted not only excess epinephrine but also norepinephrine, the effector hormone of the sympathetic nervous system. While excess activity of the sympathetic nervous system is believed to be present in TAB by most investigators who have studied this disorder, it has only recently been suspected (Fukudo et al., 1992) that possibly a diminished activity of the parasympathetic nervous system may occur in this disorder.

THE HORMONAL DYSFUNCTIONS OF TAB

Excess Discharge of Norepinephrine and Epinephrine

I already have alluded to the excess discharge of norepinephrine in TAB subjects. This hormone, synthesized by the terminal branches of the sympathetic nervous system, serves as the effector hormone of the sympathetic nervous system by which the latter effects its multifarious activities in the body. Although scientists are reasonably cognizant of the cardiovascular functions of norepinephrine (including its vasoconstrictor as well as vasodilator actions), we have much to learn about this hormone's direct role in the metabolism of various organs of the body, including the brain. When one considers the widespread employment today of drugs that block the artery-narrowing activities of norepinephrine, one cannot help but be impressed by the importance of this hormone, whose actual existence, much less its measurement, was unknown before the 1930s.

Epinephrine, unlike norepinephrine, has been recognized as an adrenal-synthesized hormone before the advent of this century. Although its increased secretion has been observed in the TAB syndrome, it is a hormone that is far more likely to be discharged by a person overtaken by fear than by a person engaged in a struggle. In short, whereas a clenched hand might serve as a logo for excess secretion of norepinephrine, a trembling hand might be an appropriate symbol for excess secretion of epinephrine.

Possible Decreased Secretion of Acetylcholine

As far as I know, no group of investigators has demonstrated an actual decreased secretion of acetylcholine at the terminal segments of the parasympathetic nervous system, although the pharmacological studies of Fukudo (Fukudo et al., 1992) suggest the possibility of such decreased parasympathetic discharge of acetylcholine.

It is my opinion, however, that even if a diminished secretion of acetylcholine occurs in TAB, such derangement plays little or no role in the pathogenesis of the disorders now strongly suspected of being related to TAB.

Excess Discharge of Adrenocorticotrophic Hormone

The pituitary gland has long been known to discharge an increased amount of adrenocorticotrophic hormone (ACTH) following stress of any kind. That is why my associates and I, early in our TAB investigations, suspected that the pituitary discharge of ACTH was increased in a significant fraction. Another reason was our clinical observation that a significant number of TAB subjects display a permanent brown deposit in their eyelids that we have described as periorbital pigmentation. Increased secretion of ACTH (as occurs, for example, in Addison's disease) is well known to lead to such deposits of melanin, which is responsible for the brown pigmentation of the eyelids.

Actual proof of an increased secretion of ACTH in TAB, however, occurred when we measured, with the cooperation of Rosalyn Yalow, the blood ACTH level of both type A and type B subjects. My associates and I (Friedman, Byers, & Rosenman, 1972) found that the average level of this hormone was significantly higher in the type A than the type B subjects throughout the day. Indirect confirmation of such excess discharge of ACTH was obtained by Williams and co-workers (1982) that their type A subjects secreted more cortisone than their type B subjects—a phenomenon presupposing an increased secretion of the adrenal-stimulating ACTH.

Excess Secretion of Testosterone

Excess secretion of testosterone was observed in type A subjects independently by both Williams and co-workers (1982) and Zumoff and co-workers (1984). Precisely what role this excess secretion of this male hormone might play in the pathogenesis of coronary heart disease remains unknown.

Decreased Serum Concentration of Growth Hormone

Unlike the other hormones affected by TAB (with the possible exception of acetylcholine), the secretion of pituitary growth hormone in most subjects with TAB is either decreased or its rate of catabolism or excretion is abnormally increased (Dreyfuss & Czazkes, 1959). Whatever may be the mechanism at play, the serum level of this hormone is reduced in the majority of TAB patients.

The reduced level of growth hormone in this disorder may be of more importance than generally is recognized because few investigators studying the causes of hypercholesterolemia appear cognizant of the role of pituitary growth hormone in the metabolism and blood level concentrations of this same sterol (Friedman & Rosenman, 1974).

ABNORMAL METABOLISM OF CHOLESTEROL AND TRIGLYCERIDES

Hypercholesterolemia

Elevated blood levels of cholesterol (hypercholesterolemia) have been attributed to such various causes as excessive intake of dietary cholesterol,

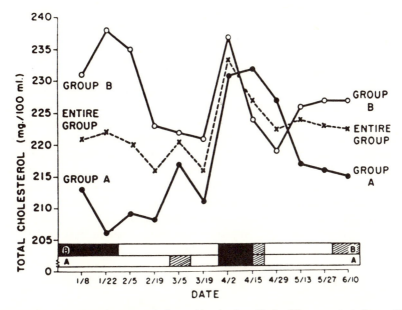

Figure 1.1. The biweekly serum cholesterol levels of certified public accountants (group B) and public accountants (group A) from January 8 to June 10. Periods of severe work stress for either group are indicated by black blocks and periods of emotional stress due to other causes than that of work by diagonally lined blocks. Note that the average serum cholesterol level of both groups rose significantly during the April 15 tax deadline period. The average serum cholesterol level rose also for the certified public accountants in early January, at which time they were stressed by inventory tasks. The public accountants were not employed for this latter function. (From Friedman et al., 1958. Reproduced with permission of *Circulation*.)

saturated fats, hypothyroidism, decreased cellular cholesterol receptor activity, and the previously mentioned inadequate blood concentration of growth hormone. However, not until 1958 was emotional stress found to effect a rise in the serum cholesterol of man (Friedman et al., 1958) (see Fig. 1.1).

Although this stress-induced phenomenon has been repeatedly confirmed (Dreyfuss & Czazkes, 1959; Gill et al., 1985; Grundy & Griffin, 1959a, b; Westlake, Wilcox, Haley, & Peterson, 1959), the average cardiologist still appears either unaware of or reluctant to believe in this mind–blood cholesterol relationship. He or she too often believes that the blood cholesterol level depends solely on what his patients ingest.

A word of caution, however; Not all TAB subjects exhibit hypercholesterolemia. Many may possess a normal or even quite low serum cholesterol concentration. On the other hand, it has been my experience that almost all persons who do exhibit hypercholesterolemia also possess TAB. The hypercholesterolemia possessed by TAB patients, of course, can usually be lowered by dietary or drug regimens, but it also can be lowered by alteration of their TAB.

The actual cause(s) responsible for the hypercholesterolemia that so frequently occurs in TAB remains to be critically elucidated. I suspect that just as changes in the distribution of blood occur in struggling animals, similar changes take place in a TAB person struggling against time, other persons, or both. Such changes, mediated by the sympathetic nervous system, result in more blood flowing to the brain and muscle and, correspondingly, less to the gastrointestinal tract, including the liver. It is my belief that this chronic reduced flow of blood to the liver may induce a change in the liver's processing of cholesterol (coming from both dietary and endogenous sources). Any such interference might well lead to an excess accumulation of cholesterol in the blood.

Hypertriglyceridemia

Here again, not all TAB subjects exhibit a high serum level of fat (i.e., hypertriglyceridemia) under fasting or after a fat-rich meal. But when a group of severely afflicted TAB persons is compared with a group of type B subjects, the TAB subjects always exhibit significantly higher average fasting as well as postprandial serum triglyceride levels (Friedman, Byers, & Rosenman, 1965; Friedman, Rosenman, & Byers, 1964). Moreover, although a small fraction of such Type A subjects may not show a higher fasting or postprandial serum triglyceride level, very rarely does a type B subject exhibit either a high fasting (i.e., above 110 mg%) or postprandial (i.e., above 140 mg%) serum concentration of triglyceride. We also found that not only did the serum triglyceride of the TAB subjects reach a peak concentration 4 hours after ingestion of a fatty meal that was twice that of the type B subjects (see Figs. 1.2 and 1.3), but at 24 hours it also remained even greater than the 4-hour postprandial peak serum content of the type B men.

This delayed removal of dietary-derived fat or triglyceride and its accumulation in the blood in the majority of severely afflicted type A subjects probably is caused by the same norepinephrine-induced hepatic ischemia and resultant dysfunction that we suspect is responsible for the hypercholesterolemia also observed in these same individuals.

Hundreds of epidemiological and psychological studies of TAB have been performed in the 35 years since the nature of and the possible coronary

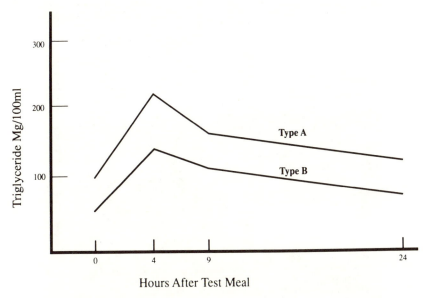

Figure 1.2. The serum triglyceride levels in types A and B men 4, 9, and 24 hours after ingestion of a standard excess triglyceride meal. Note that even 24 hours after ingestion of this single triglyceride-rich meal, the serum triglyceride level of the type A participants is greater than the 4-hour peak level of the type B subjects.

heart disease relationship of TAB were first described. However, I am not cognizant of a single attempted replication of the 1964–1967 observations (Friedman et al., 1965) concerning the hypertriglyceridemia exhibited by a significant number of TAB subjects upon ingestion of either animal or vegetable fats.

This failure to explore in depth the cause(s) of this hyperlipemic phenomenon seems tragic in view of the fact that Heberden, on first describing angina in 1772 (Heberden, 1772), called attention to its occurrence after a heavy meal. Mackenzie, later in 1923 (MacKenzie, 1923), observed that the majority of his coronary patients suffered angina after ingestion of food. Osler also (1897) certainly was aware of the danger of a heavy meal to coronary patients, because in 1897 he wrote, ". . . there is death in the pot for coronary patients." Too much contemporary preoccupation with cholesterol, and in what form it travels in blood, has obscured

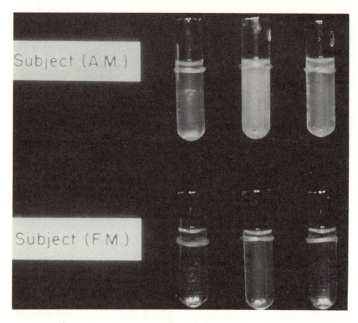

Figure 1.3. The three serum samples of a type A (top) and type B (bottom) subject before and 4 and 9 hours, respectively, after a triglyceride-rich meal.

the acute lethality of a single fat-rich meal, whether the fat is lard or safflower oil.

Postprandial Intravascular Aggregation of Erythrocytes

Knisely and associates (1947), in a special review in *Science*, described the intravascular aggregation or agglutination of erythrocytes (red blood cells) they observed on microscopic scrutiny of the small arteries and arterioles of the bulbar conjunctiva of the eyes in 600 human subjects suffering from scores of different illnesses varying from hysteria to whooping cough. Fifteen of their 600 patients suffered from coronary heart disease and all exhibited erythrocyte agglutination (which the investigators designated as "sludging").

The authors, however, claimed that they never observed this sludging process in a normal, healthy subject. They also pointed out that these clumps of erythrocytes frequently completely obstructed the flow of blood in many small arteries (arterioles), which led to the inadequate flow of

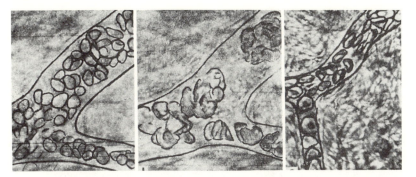

Figure 1.4.   The first diagram shows erythrocytes moving in a normal manner through a capillary. The middle diagram depicts the aggregation (sludging) of the erythrocytes 4 hours after the ingestion of a triglyceride-rich meal. The third diagram demonstrates a disappearance of the aggregation (sludging) of erythrocytes 9 hours after the ingestion of the triglyceride-rich meal.

blood to various tissues customarily nourished by these very small blood vessels. Strangely, however, they did not discuss the effect such sludging and its obstruction of blood flow might have on the small collateral vessels developing in the wake of human atherosclerosis and thrombosis in a major coronary artery. The authors also did not report any observed relationship between sludging and the blood concentration of triglyceride. Finally, because the TAB disorder was not described until a decade after these sludging studies had been done, a relationship between sludging and emotional stress was not investigated.

However, my associates and I (Friedman et al., 1965) found that TAB subjects and, in particular, coronary patients can lag in their blood clearance of ingested triglycerides (see Figs. 1.2 and 1.3) and, as a result, exhibit artery-obstructing masses of aggregated erythrocytes (see Figs. 1.4–1.6). The presently tardy recognition of these potentially lethal phenomena is due to the difficulty in observing the *in vivo* agglutination of erythrocytes. My associates and I (Friedman et al., 1964) were able to do so by magnifying and photographing the small arterioles of the bulbar conjunctiva (see Figs. 1.4–1.6). This difficulty in observing fat-induced agglutination of erythrocytes is the reason that this phenomenon presently is not in the paradigm of cardiovascular pathology. But it is probably the major reason that just a single, heavy fat meal may be lethal. Conversely, it is probably the reason that persons with stable angina become free of it within several days of a fat-free diet. Apparently, such a diet prevents the clumping of erythrocytes

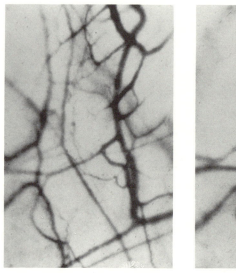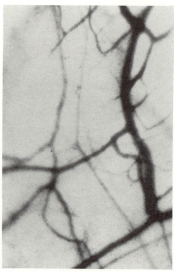

Figure 1.5. Photographs of conjunctival arterioles of a type B subject before (left) and 4 hours after (right) the ingestion of a triglyceride-rich meal. Note the absence of sludging of erythrocytes in both photographs. (From Friedman et al., 1965. Reproduced with permission.)

that previously led to an obstruction in the blood flow of the tiny collateral blood vessels of the heart.

TYPE B BEHAVIOR

Hormonal Functions in Type B Behavior

The type B behavior (TBB) person exhibits none of the hormonal dysfunctions observed in TAB subjects. Thus, my associates and I (Friedman et al., 1960) have found that their blood levels as well as their rate of urinary excretion of norepinephrine are normal. Likewise, their blood levels of ACTH (Friedman et al., 1972) and urinary excretion of testosterone (Zumoff et al., 1984) are normal.

As a result of these normal hormonal secretions, the blood cholesterol and triglyceride concentrations of TBB participants are rarely elevated (Friedman & Rosenman, 1974; Friedman et al., 1964). Because of their

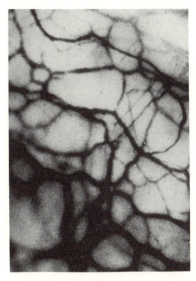 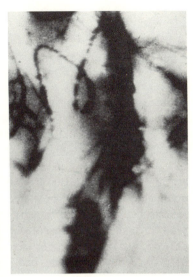

Figure 1.6. Photographs of conjunctival arterioles of a type A subject before (left) and 4 hours after (right) the ingestion of a triglyceride-rich meal. Note the marked sludging of erythrocyte and resultant "beading" and interruption of flow in the arterioles 4 hours after the ingestion of the triglyceride-rich meal.

normal rapid disposition of dietary triglycerides, the agglutination or sludging of erythrocytes is rarely seen in TBB subjects.

The Psychological Characteristics of TBB

The fundamental characteristic and bulwark of the TBB are its components of adequate security and self-esteem. The TBB person's possession of these two emotional qualities is what most sharply differentiates the TBB from the TAB person. The TBB person is a well person because he or she feels secure and enjoys sufficient self-esteem. The TAB person is unwell because he or she does not feel secure or does not possess sufficient self-esteem.

Probably because of feeling secure and esteeming himself or herself sufficiently, the TBB person possesses the following abilities:

1. He or she can give love and affection as well as accept it. The TBB person, unlike the TAB person, almost always received in his or her early childhood sufficient (i.e., unconditional) affection, love, and admiration

from both his or her parents. And more often than not, these parental feelings were articulated. In turn, he or she found it relatively easy to express his or her own love and admiration for his or her parents. Because of this early reception and giving of love and admiration, the TBB person naturally is capable of giving and receiving these important emotional attributes to other persons.

2. He or she can tolerate, without becoming irritated or hostile, the trivial or venial errors of commission or omission of other individuals. The TBB person recognizes that everyone, including himself or herself, makes mistakes or errors. He or she also knows that a mistake that is made and corrected often serves as an excellent learning experience. This tolerance of the TBB person also extends to his or her social intercourse. He or she finds no need to attempt to bolster his or her self-esteem by correcting the grammatical or pronunciatory errors of his or her friends or acquaintants. Nor will he or she brusquely correct his or her friends or acquaintants if they do not report correctly or exactly some petty fact or happening. In short, he or she rarely becomes captious in casual, social intercourse of any kind.

3. He or she rarely indulges in conversational proleptic behavior. The TBB individual recognizes that his or her family members, friends, and acquaintances deserve the privilege and courtesy of finishing their own sentences in which they present their views, descriptions, and deductions without anticipatory verbal foreclosure.

4. He or she can listen to others without impatience. While the TAB person often finds it difficult to listen to the speech of others, particularly his or her peers and subordinates, the TBB person knows that often the speech of others can be useful, instructive and sometimes even relaxation inducing. He or she also avoids any attempt to hasten the speech of others. This quality, however, does not prevent him or her from politely but decisively terminating the speech of persons who are not his or her vocational superiors but whose conversations are boring, banal, or needlessly pleonastic.

5. He or she can accept with composure not only constructive but also destructive criticism. As I shall discuss in a subsequent chapter, the TAB person finds it difficult to translate any praise he or she may receive into enhancement of his or her self-esteem. However, he or she can be devastated by criticism, even if such criticism is constructive and helpful. Quite to the contrary, the TBB person accepts criticism as a learning process, bearing no direct connection whatsoever with either his or her security or self-esteem. While not finding destructive criticism pleasing, again he or she searches for the possible aid even this form of criticism may provide.

6. He or she finds no difficulty, when necessary, in delegating work to others. The late president of Yale University, Kingman Brewster, once remarked, "Truly effective delegation does not consist of assigning only trivial tasks to a subordinate but also to assign moderately important responsibilities *and be willing to take the responsibility that the subordinate may err in the execution of the assignment*" (personal communication, 1977). The TBB subject's sense of security is stable enough for him or her to take this moderate risk. He or she will step in to correct a delegated procedure being wrongly executed only if the error will lead to serious or irretrievable damage to himself or herself or his or her organization.

7. He or she finds it reasonably easy to trust others. Secretary of War, Henry Stimson, at age 78, once wrote a memorandum (9/11/45) to President Truman in which he said, "The chief lesson I have learned in a long life is that the only way you make a man trustworthy is to trust him and the surest way to make him untrustworthy is to distrust him and show your distrust." The TBB person, always aware of his or her own integrity, naturally enough believes that most other people possess integrity. He or she, of course, knows that occasionally he or she may be cheated or maligned, but feels this is a moderately modest price to pay to avoid creating a lifelong ambience in which evil predominates.

8. He or she attempts to avoid excessive egoism and egocentrism. The TBB person almost instinctively shies away from employing too often the first person singular pronoun in his or her speech. In this connection, Scherwitz (1986) observed in the MRFIT Study that subjects who at entry employed the first person singular pronoun in their interviews subsequently suffered coronary artery disease significantly more frequently than those volunteers who escaped suffering a later coronary accident.

Also, the TBB person, while not necessarily avoiding discussing subjects in which he or she is involved or interested in, is quite capable of becoming interested in and discussing matters in which he or she has not, is not, and will not be involved. Such diversion is not easy for the TAB person to perform.

9. He or she attempts to retain all facets of his or her personality. Although there are exceptions, the majority of TBB persons attempt to maintain the contours of the personality they possessed in their late adolescence and early adulthood. During this period of their lives, most of them became interested not only in indulging and watching sports, attending the cinema, and engaging in various social activities, but also in becoming acquainted, at least, with the humanities.

In short, the average TBB person, as he or she advances into middle age, continues to take an interest in many of the activities and subjects that he or she earlier had enjoyed. Numerical affairs might, as he or she ages, require much of his or her attention, but not at the expense of a total erosion of his or her numinous entities. His or her right-brain activities have not been preempted by the oppressive domination of his or her left-brain activities of calculating, enumerating, and accumulating diverse data.

10. He or she can easily afford to laugh at himself or herself. The TBB person possesses a truly good sense of humor in that he or she is able to see himself or herself as all of us should see ourselves sometimes, namely, preposterous or quixotic. He or she recognizes that to be able to sometimes laugh at himself or herself is a fine way to bring balance and perspective into his or her life.

11. He or she is able to find time both to meditate about the goals and purposes of his or her life and to remember his or her past. Loren Eisely (1969) wrote, "Beware the mind-destroying drug of constant action." Just as creative thinking cannot easily be accomplished by a cyclist pedaling at a breakneck speed, neither can it be accomplished by a person figuratively pedaling furiously through every day of his life. The basic concept leading to the development of the laser beam did not come to TBB Nobel Laureate Charles Townes while he was running to catch a Washington bus, but while he was sitting on a Washington park bench staring almost absentmindedly at an azalea bush in full red bloom. To this day, he does not know why or how the red blossoms gave birth to his awesome creation, the laser beam. He only is certain that he was just meditating in the park (personal statement).

This last anecdote does not imply that all TBB scientists possess the potential of becoming Nobel laureates or that all Nobel laureate scientists are TBB individuals. But it does suggest that time taken for meditation or contemplation is not inimical to creative thinking.

It is, however, the capability of the TBB person to recollect periodically and regularly his or her past achievements and happiness that pleasantly seasons his or her outlook for the future. It is this particular habit of drawing sustenance from the past that helps support his or her relatively high degree of self-esteem and confidence that whatever future contingencies he or she may encounter, he or she will be able to cope with them. This is a confidence not usually observed in the TAB subject.

12. He or she does not suffer from either a sense of time urgency or impatience. The TBB person avoids suffering from a sense of time urgency and its frequent sequential congener, hostility, simply because he or she infrequently feels any necessity of attempting to achieve or acquire too many things in too little time. He or she also avoids attempting to participate in too many activities.

Simply stated, the TBB person either instinctively recognizes or has learned how to recognize the limits of any given paradigm of time available for the execution of one or a related series of activities, and he or she does not struggle against these limits. This is a simple bit of logic that the TAB person either has never learned or has forgotten. Thus, in a peculiar sort of way, the TBB person never thinks of time as an enemy but as a friend; the TAB person almost never can achieve this sort of friendship.

13. He does not suffer from free-floating hostility. As already repeatedly emphasized, TAB subjects, because of their inadequate self-esteem, easily react hostilely to what they consider the thoughtless or heinous acts of other people. The adequate self-esteem, however, of the TBB person shields him or her from intrusions of hostility. This being so, when he or she encounters minor misdemeanors of others, he or she is quite apt to overlook, to feel compassion for, or to forgive their actions. He or she demonstrates a very simple psychological truth: When one is content with one's self, it is easy to overlook the trivial faults of others.

However, the TBB individual by no means is a "Casper Milquetoast." Confronted with a grievous, uncalled-for act of malevolence or evil, he or she will take the appropriate measures to defend himself or herself. He or she just does not explode with a burst of hostility if he or she encounters such activities as a person carrying 12 or 13, instead of less than 10, grocery items in the express lane of a supermarket or a motorist following him too closely on a freeway.

All the previous qualities and abilities of the TBB subject have received almost no attention from the hundreds of investigators who have interested themselves in TAB. However, recently Kaplan (1992), in a totally charming and perceptive manner, has given his description of what a type B person is. It deserves the attention of any person interested in the TAB problem.

I shall end this section by inserting a letter sent to an old TBB parent by his middle-aged son who had the opportunity of observing his father for over 40 years.

A Short List of the Things I Most Love about My Father

1. His consistent and unflagging devotion to family—the spirit of Dickens' *Christmas Carol* practiced every day, throughout the year; especially love of children and grandchildren.

2. His values—including extraordinary self-discipline and work ethic, i.e, the willingness to accept "short-term pain for long-term gain."

3. The value of financial/fiscal conservation over superficial or "conspicuous" wealth or possessions.

4. The love, respect, and enjoyment of knowledge, purely for its own sake, including the wonderful companionship that good books and an eclectic library alone provide.

5. Dedication and cultivation of friendships—taking the time and effort to maintain close friendships—rewarded by the love and respect of many, many fine and wonderful friends, colleagues, and "fans."

6. Love and appreciation of fine books, art, flora, and the simple pleasures of family life; a trip to the nursery, an art gallery, or, on occasion, a Florentine chapel or London bookshop.

7. The willingness to forgive the faults of others, and a humble and self-effacing opinion of his own talent and ability.

8. A joyful, playful, and lighthearted ability to interact with children, friends, the family pets, and life in general, including the difficult art of being able to laugh at himself.

9. The undaunted and undiminished willingness, even at age 70, to interact vigorously and joyfully with life, work, friends, clubs, travel, and family. (No more "floating rest home" Chesapeake Bay cruises for this "senior citizen!")

10. The willingness to accept, live with, and accommodate the difficulties, trials, and challenges that long-term lives, marriages, careers, and relationships inevitably place before us.

TAB IN WOMEN

The prevalence of TAB in women probably cannot ever be determined with accuracy. This is because the type and character of the group of women will greatly affect the prevalence of TAB. For example, the women of a well-developed country undoubtedly will have a profoundly different TAB prevalence than that shown by women of a Third World nation. Even in the United States, it is highly unlikely that the TAB prevalence in women working in the offices of Manhattan will be similar to that observed in farming housewives in the general vicinity of the Amish village Intercourse in Pennsylvania.

There are, however, some published reports describing the TAB prevalence in American groups of women. Moss and associates (1986), employing the structured interview as their diagnostic instrument, found that the prevalence of TAB was as great (64%) in the women as in the men they studied. Chesney, Black, Frautschi, and De Busk (1986) observed that the prevalence of TAB was significantly less in housewives than in working women.

My own studies have focused chiefly on volunteers from commerce and industry, most of whom have been males. Consequently, I am not able to estimate accurately the prevalence of TAB in women. I agree, however, with the belief of Thoresen and Low (1990) that the prevalence of TAB in the total American women population probably lies in the 50–60% range.

Relationship of TAB and Coronary Heart Disease in Women

Haynes, Feinleib, Levine, Scotch, and Kannel (1980) observed that a sizable number of women in the Framingham Study were found to possess TAB. These women, when followed for 8 years, were found to suffer significantly more frequently from angina (but not infarctions) than the initially assessed TBB women. When this same group of Framingham women was reexamined 14 years later by a new set of investigators (Eaker & Castelli, 1988), the TAB women again were found to suffer significantly more frequently from angina (but not infarction) than the TBB women.*

Most other investigators (Blumenthal, Williams, Kong, Shanberg, & Thompson, 1978; Frank, Heller, Kornfeld, Sporn, & Weiss, 1976) also have reported that TAB women appeared to harbor more coronary atherosclerosis. More recently, however, Powell et al. (1993), studying the six deaths in the women of our Recurrent Coronary Prevention Project (RCPP) (Friedman et al., 1986), hypothesized that postinfarction women who exhibited less severe TAB were more apt to suffer a cardiac death than more severely afflicted TAB postinfarction women. Unfortunately, the authors made a simple arithmetical error in their study that subverted the integrity of their hypotheses. Certainly at entrance into the RCPP study (Friedman et al., 1986), postmyocardial women without exception exhibited moderate to severe TAB. Stated in a slightly different manner, I can declare that although women suffer significantly fewer infarctions, when one does suffer from this cardiac catastrophe, she invariably also has suffered from TAB, although she often attempts to hide its hostility component.

---

*It is puzzling that this second set of Framingham investigators, while confirming the earlier findings that significantly more angina occurred in the TAB women, nevertheless in the summary of their article substitute the vague phrase "pain in a woman's chest" for the angina pectoris that had been diagnosed.

THE COVERT AND OVERT COMPONENTS OF TAB

Insecurity and Inadequate Self-Esteem and Its Causes

Despite the primary role this covert component (insecurity/inadequate self-esteem) almost invariably plays in the pathogenesis of TAB, my associates and I were not aware of either its existence or its causal role in the disorder during the first decade of our research studies of TAB subjects. Even at the present time, only a few TAB investigators (Gatson & Teevan, 1980; Houston & Kelly, 1987; Houston & Vavack, 1991; Price et al., 1995) are aware of its overriding importance in this syndrome.

My colleagues and I were tardy in detecting its presence in TAB subjects primarily because it was difficult for us to perceive from our initial encounters with these subjects, so many of whom were seemingly very self-assured and self-confident, that they all harbored a core of insecurity/inadequate self-esteem. But when we began counseling TAB patients, it did not take many therapy sessions before we, and also they, recognized the presence of this component.

Origin of Insecurity and Inadequate Self-Esteem in Childhood and Adolescence

The inadequate self-esteem phase of this component in the majority of cases begins quite early in childhood and seemingly arises because of the perceived absence of sufficient *expressed* affection and admiration from both parents. Here are some of the statements made by some of our TAB participants, all of whom were over 45 years of age:

1. "I don't remember my mother ever hugging or kissing me."
2. "If I brought home a report card with just one B on it and all the rest A grades, I still was treated like a criminal."
3. "My younger brother was my father's favorite. He was Jacob and I was Esau."
4. "When I told my father I was chosen as an All-American basketball player, all he said was, 'Well, I still think your brother is a better player.' And when he said that, that was it. I just gave up because I knew I could never make his team. I never talked to him again."
5. "When I sometimes quarreled or fought with my brothers or sisters, they were never disciplined, only I received their censure or punishment."

We asked 110 TAB coronary patients to answer anonymously two questions: (1) Did they receive sufficient affection and admiration in childhood from both their parents? (2) At what age did their free-floating hostility begin? Seventy of the 110 (64%) responded that they did not receive sufficient affection and admiration. It was of interest that of these 70 patients, 51 (73%) also declared that their free-floating hostility began before the age of 10. In this last particular, of the 40 patients who responded that they had received adequate affection and admiration from both patients, only three (8%) reported that their free-floating hostility began before the age of 10.

But as our anonymous inquiry revealed, the inadequate self-esteem of TAB by no means always begins and springs solely from insufficient parental fondness and appreciation. It may and frequently does arise in the elementary, high school, college, or later periods in the lives of TAB participants. For example, a 55-year-old TAB participant, insisting that he had received quite adequate love, admiration, and respect from his mother and father, wrote recently to us:

> My inadequate self-esteem began when I was 7 years of age. It began one day when my second grade teacher and my fellow students laughed at my inability to read a sentence in class. After they laughed at me, I stopped trying to read. Superiority in arithmetic became my goal to conquer (and an "I'll show them" attitude). Listening and math skills developed while reading and writing lay dormant. Hostilities, due to my reading difficulties, continue to this day.

Compensatory Attempts to Substitute for Absence of Biparental Affection and Admiration

When inadequate self-esteem begins, as it appears to do in most cases because of insufficient biparental devotion, the affected child usually attempts to compensate for this perceived absence by seeking emotional enhancement outside the home and family circle. But in seeking emotional substitutes, the child does not seek love or affection from his or her contemporaries but rather he or she strives for their respect, admiration, and often their envy. To accomplish these ends, the child attempts to achieve and to acquire more things than his or her contemporaries. In short, the child believes he or she can enhance his or her damaged sense of self-esteem by seeing to it that the ratio or achievements versus expectations never falls below unity.

But accumulation of things, no matter how quantitatively impressive it may become, never succeeds in appeasing the ever-increasing expectations of the TAB subject. This is in great part due to his or her failure from the very beginning to include in his or her category of expectations a capacity not only to receive and to give affection but to evaluate it increasingly more than his or her often frenetic amassment of things and power.

Even the achievement by a TAB sufferer of the presidency of his or her company, the acquisition of a second or third glamorous spouse, the ownership of several or more elegant homes, and the accumulation of a half-dozen top-of-the-line automobiles may be significant achievements, but by themselves they cannot appease the still-present longing for the affection and admiration that this TAB sufferer did not receive in his or her childhood from his or her parents. Almost paradoxically, these dazzling but worldly accomplishments and acquisitions might worsen his or her underlying sense of inadequate self-esteem.

Continuous Apprehension of Future Contingencies

Perhaps one of the most uncomfortable feelings emanating from the presence of the insecurity/inadequate self-esteem of TAB individuals is their constant apprehension of future disasters that they may encounter. This feeling persists even when such a person has just secured a triumph. For example, one of our TAB participants, the president of a large corporation, told us that he did not enjoy a dinner party with his senior executives celebrating a 34% increase in annual profits because he kept thinking that possibly the corporation might experience lesser or even no profits in the forthcoming year. No therapist who has counseled TAB individuals can escape the conclusion that while such persons can easily manage exigencies, they live in dread of possible contingencies. The insecurity and inadequate self-esteem of the TAB person in the absence of effective counseling may progressively worsen so that he or she feels unnaturally depressed if he or she fails to win at any contest, whether it is a game of tennis or golf with a friend or even a game of Ping-Pong with an adolescent daughter or son.

Extreme Sensitivity to Criticism and Relative Nonresponsiveness to Praise

Another aspect of the TAB subject's self-esteem is its tendency to worsen on receipt of the slightest criticism by other persons but, conversely, its failure to be enhanced by the praise or rewards offered by friends or even institutions. For example, a very distinguished TAB scientist confessed to us that while he was being awarded a most prestigious medal and a standing ovation by his eminent colleagues following the presentation, he found himself unmoved and impatiently awaiting the end of the ceremony. "I later wondered for quite a while why I was so unmoved during this event and the only reason I could come up with was that it would have meant something to me if either of my parents had still been alive and present when I was awarded the prize."

Finally, it is the insecurity and inadequate self-esteem that encourages the emergence of free-floating hostility in the TAB person. It is very difficult to find other individuals praiseworthy until one learns to believe that he or she, too, is praiseworthy.

Relationship of Anxiety and Depression to Insecurity/Inadequate Self-Esteem

Insecurity/inadequate self-esteem, if severe enough and if not adequately compensated for, also can and frequently does play a very significant role in initiating and sustaining an anxiety state or depression. The therapist thus may sometimes be in a quandary on how to differentiate TAB from either of these two other emotional states.

Ordinarily, the TAB person from the very beginning attempts to compensate for or combat his or her incipient anxiety or even depression by indulging somewhat ceaselessly in activities of accomplishment or accumulation. These latter activities hide from his or her consciousness the deeply entrenched and quiescent insecurity/inadequate self-esteem.

Conversely, the person who lacks the energy to indulge in various activities that may distract him/her from a deep-seated state of insecurity/inadequate self-esteem may well develop a state of anxiety or even depression. It is not far from the truth that when a TAB person encounters a chronically anxious or depressed person, he or she might say, "There but for the grace of effort, go I."

2

Psychological Components of Type A Behavior

TIME URGENCY/IMPATIENCE

Time urgency is, as I shall demonstrate in Chapter 3, the major overt type A behavior (TAB) component. It is essentially a persistent feeling the TAB person has that there is not or will not be sufficient time to accomplish the things that he or she feels should be done.

This temporal tension very frequently, indeed almost invariably, deteriorates to a variant of hostility (i.e., irascibility or irritability) if the TAB person becomes increasingly frustrated at not being able to achieve his or her goals in the available time span.

During the past decade, a number of investigators employing self-report questionnaires and multivariate analysis as their instruments to determine which of the two TAB overt manifestations might be the most coronary-prone risk factor have concluded that the TAB hostility component is the "toxic" agent and that the time urgency/impatience component is essentially harmless. The tragic error in freeing time urgency of coronary complicity will be discussed in Chapter 3. Suffice it to say that the time urgency/impatience component is as fully or even more involved than the hostility component in the premature onset of coronary heart disease.

THE CAUSES OF TIME URGENCY/IMPATIENCE

Covert Insecurity/Inadequate Self-Esteem

As already stated, the time-urgent person almost always harbors a feeling of insecurity or inadequate self-esteem. Because of this underlying emotional inadequacy, the person suffering from it tries to ameliorate its persistent, nagging perturbation by attempting to acquire as many achievements or to engage in as many activities as he or she possibly can. But far too often, the quality of the achievements and activities give way to mere quantity. Because of this increasing qualitative triviality of both achievements and activities, the underlying insecurity or inadequate self-esteem is not lessened but increased. This leads to a vicious and endless circle in which the sense of time urgency worsens.

A common enough example of this transmogrification of the quality of one's achievements to that of quantification is presented by an initially superb novelist who, driven by his or her insecurity, hurriedly writes and publishes an increasing number of essentially vapid books. A similar example is a scientist who, undermined by his or her insecurity, opts to involve himself in a number of trivial studies that are certain of publication rather than tackle a truly significant problem whose time for successful resolution may be indefinite.

The Cult of Speed

I have discussed in considerable detail in Chapter 1 the cultivation of speed in almost all our societal, industrial, and professional activities. It is my belief that this societal cultivation of haste is one of the major causes of time urgency.

Greed

Greed as a cause of time urgency admittedly is not a pleasant topic to discuss, but oversight of its presence in a person suffering from time urgency does not lead to its spontaneous disappearance. Greed capable of intensifying a sense of time urgency may be sheer avarice (i.e., an excessive, reprehensible acquisition for too many things) or an inordinate drive to participate in too many events. Although a facile excuse for either type of greed can be attributed to a basic insecurity, it is also quite possible that greed sometimes, particularly greed concerned with excessive acquisition of things, may spring from factors other than a basic insecurity defect.

Chronic Failure to Refrain from Giving Excess, Time-Consuming Aid to Other Persons or Organizations

Today, business and professional leaders of a community are expected to lend a helping hand to the multiple organizations of that same community. Even a business executive of just moderate economic status might be asked to coach or otherwise participate in his or her community's Little League baseball. Other executives might be asked to serve as active members of the board of trustees of their church or service club, as well as participate in additional diverse community services.

But if there is to be a reasonable amount of leisure, relaxation, and participation in the activities of one's own family, that person must put a limit to excess participation in community activities. However, because so often the type A person exhibits a facial and vocal sense of determination and decision, he or she is considered an excellent candidate for leadership and participation in the myriad community activities now extant, and so he or she is especially importuned for these activities.

Unfortunately, too many TAB persons, wishing to be well liked at all costs, find it extraordinarily difficult to refuse such requests. As a consequence of these multiple involvements, he or she finds that time is no longer his or her friend but an implacable enemy. Hence, a sense of time urgency is born or enhanced.

Failure in Process of Delegation

Because of the underlying persistent insecurity of so many TAB subjects, they find it difficult to delegate to their peers (and especially their subordinates) various tasks and activities that must be done and that these persons are usually as capable of accomplishing despite the doubts of TAB individuals.

Needless Self-Imposition of Deadlines

A not infrequent cause of time urgency in TAB subjects is their inveterate tendency to set definite dates at which various activities should be accomplished, neglecting to take into full consideration the possible delaying effects of various contingencies not considered when a completion date is declared.

FREE-FLOATING HOSTILITY

Dysfunctional Family Relationships

There are few TAB subjects afflicted with moderate to severe free-floating hostility who do not experience familial difficulties. Such difficulties involve both the spouses and the children. The most frequent emotional manifestation of the TAB person's free-floating hostility is his or her increasing failure to verbalize frank and frequent affection and admiration for his or her spouse. In its place, he or she substitutes competition and rivalry and an increasing criticism of the domestic activities of the spouse.

The competition takes place in any marital activity including sports, card games, and even in skirmishes for conversational dominance. Since almost all spouses of TAB persons also possess type A behavior, it is easy to understand that marital contests and conflicts, whether they are games of tennis, golf, bridge, or dominoes, often can become rancorous although the contestants may not overtly reveal their discomfiture. For example, it is often common for TAB spouses to keep continuing secret day-by-day scores of victories in their contests with each other.

In addition to this consummate desire to win in all marital contests, the TAB person comes into conflict with his or her spouse concerning even trivial domestic activities. For example, a TAB person frequently argues with his or her spouse about (1) the correct method of installing a roll of toilet paper so that it unwinds in the direction he or she believes is proper, (2) the correct way of hanging his or her clothes, (3) the correct temperature of the home, (4) the choice of a television program, (5) the wattage of light bulbs, (6) the choice and preparation of the food that is served at dinners, and last but not least, (7) the discipline and instruction of the children. As one of our TAB participants admitted, "Each evening before I open our front door, I review the things I want to complain about."

The relationship of the TAB person with his or her children often suffers not only from his or her own desire to win in all contests with them, but also for them to excel among their own contemporaries. Even when playing with their children of only 9 or 10 years of age, the male TAB person finds it exceedingly difficult to permit his child to win even a single game of checkers, dominoes, or Ping-Pong: "He or she has got to learn that to win, he or she must deserve to win. It would be dishonest if I purposely let him or her win." This is the excuse he gives for his desire to win, but the true reason for his inability to let his child ever win is that his own self-esteem is so tenuous that he strives to win at all times, regardless of the circumstances attending the contest.

On the other hand, the male type B person laughingly remarks that he sometimes lets his small son or daughter win a contest. "If I win every time, they may get discouraged and quit playing," he almost always has told us. His adequate self-esteem can withstand a defeat in checkers administered to him by his 7-year-old son or daughter.

These contests between a male TAB person and his children tend to become more intense and bitter when the children become adolescents. These strifes may become so anger-inciting that one wife of one our TAB participants has called the police to intervene.

It is not the possible animosity arising from excessive competition in games, however, that leads to the estrangement between the male TAB person and his children. It is his incessant criticism of many of their habits, actions, and attitudes of which he does not approve. He wishes them to excel in activities that he believes to be important. Unfortunately, he so often assumes the role of devastating critic that he finds it almost hypocritical to show or verbalize affection. It is as if he feels that such a display somehow might weaken his role as critic. He criticizes, be believes, not because he wishes to control the actions of his children but because he is certain that he knows what is best for them and their future. He never realizes the emotional scar he produces in their lives by failing to give them his affection and admiration.

Frequent Loss of Temper while Driving

If all motorists on the highway (1) drove at a speed that did not exceed the speed limit and yet never impeded the TAB person's own passage, (2) never cut too sharply into in his or her lane, (3) never drove too closely to the rear of his or her car, (4) never fishtailed his or her own car, and (5) meticulously obeyed all highway signals and directions, the TAB person probably would not become either angry or hostile when driving a car. But unfortunately not all persons on city streets or highways drive in this fashion. As a consequence, the TAB person who drives a car, particularly on a highway, experiences anger and hostility. Moreover, even if he or she encounters only satisfactory drivers but there is a delay in traffic, his or her impatience quickly devolves into anger.

Chronic Inability to Feel Joy at the Achievements of Others

It is difficult for a TAB person to experience exultation or even long-lasting pleasure at successes or pleasant happenings of his or her closest friends or even members of his or her own family. As we previously emphasized, even his or her own achievements or successes afford only short-lasting palliative support to his or her inadequate self-esteem.

Intolerance of Even the Trivial Errors of Omission and Commission by Others

Just as the TAB person expects perfect performance by drivers on the highway and becomes hostile if they make errors, so he or she becomes similarly disturbed when persons behave or act in a manner that he or she considers erroneous. If one of his or her subordinates misspells a word or makes a grammatical error in a memorandum, the TAB person becomes unduly irritated. Similarly, he or she becomes irascible whenever he or she believes he or she is served food by a slightly unskilled waiter or waitress or is poorly attended to by a sales associate or clerk. The TAB person also easily becomes irritated if kept waiting for more than a few minutes not only by a member of his or her family but also by anyone else, including the physician, dentist, and barber.

This easily aroused anger following any perceived breach of conduct, regardless of its nature, is the reason I describe the TAB person's hostility as free-floating. In a very real sense, it is probable that the TAB person seeks a myriad of various incitements to divert his or her covert dissatisfaction with himself or herself.

Disbelief in Altruism

It is almost impossible to believe in the good-heartedness and unselfishness of other persons if one chronically minimizes his or her own worthiness. Guilty of underevaluation of their own integrity, a certain fraction of TAB persons remain fixedly suspicious of the motives of most of the people they encounter, although they very infrequently suspect their spouse of infidelity or their children of theft or worse felonies. Nor are all TAB persons, possessing hostility, beset by the conviction that "everyone thinks only of himself and his own goals." It has been my impression that in a peculiar sense most TAB persons who are cynical are ashamed of harboring this wretched manifestation of their covert, inadequate self-esteem.

3

Medical Diagnosis of Type A Behavior and Its Differentiation from Type B Behavior

REASONS FOR THE STILL-PRESENT CONFUSION CONCERNING THE DIAGNOSIS OF TAB AND ITS RELATIONSHIP TO CORONARY HEART DISEASE

The confusion concerning the relationship of TAB to the pathogenesis of coronary heart disease has been due to two reasons. The most important has been and still is the failure of almost all investigators in the field to recognize that, despite its ubiquity in the American population [as is also coronary artery disease (Enos, Beyer, & Holmes, 1955)], TAB is a medical disorder, and like all other medical disorders, whether aquired immunodeficiency syndrome (AIDS) or acne, cannot be diagnosed by a self-report obtained by a questionnaire or by a nonprofessional clerk.

The proper detection of TAB can only be accomplished by an examination, not by an interview, not even by the so-called "gold standard" structured interview (SI). Moreover, the examination must seek not only the possible identifying symptoms and traits but also, even more importantly, the physical or psychomotor signs suggesting the presence of TAB. Finally, the examiner not only requires extensive instruction, but he or she must also possess an inherent aptitude for this particular kind of diagnosis. I emphasize this last prerequisite because in my experience I have found

31

that some psychologists, despite instruction and training, find it difficult to detect the all-important psychomotor signs of TAB.

If these criteria are needed for the proper detection of TAB, then the results of various epidemiological and clinical studies (Ahern et al., 1990; Barefoot et al., 1989; Case, Heller, Case & Moss, 1985; Ruberman, Weinblatt, Goldberg, & Chaudhary, 1984; Shekelle et al., 1985) concerned with the relationship of TAB to coronary heart disease (CHD) cannot be accepted with any degree of confidence because all TAB diagnoses in these studies were done by self-report questionnaire procedures.

A second development leading to controversy and confusion concerning the diagnosis of TAB has been the recent attempts of a number of investigators (Barefoot, Dahlstrom, & Williams, 1983; Dembroski, MacDougall, Costa, & Grandits, 1989; Williams, Haney, & Lee, 1988) to attribute coronary risk potential to only the hostility component of TAB. These investigators thus have tended to exculpate time urgency, the second TAB component, from any complicity in the pathogenesis of CHD. Once again, questionnaires and doubtful statistical dynamics were utilized to incriminate hostility and to absolve time urgency in the premature induction of CHD.

However, other investigators (Hearn, Murray, & Luepker, 1989; Helmer, Ragland, & Syme, 1991; Leon, Finn, Murray, & Bailey, 1988; Osler, 1897), again employing the same questionnaires as well as other types of self-report scales, absolve hostility completely in the pathogenesis of CHD.

What is one to conclude from these completely contradictory results? Helmer and associates (1991), in denying hostility as a risk factor, conclude that these contradictory results concerning the CHD relevance of hostility indicate the need for caution in drawing broad conclusions from the results of individual studies.

The latter warning of the need for caution proposed by these epidemiologists is all very well, but they themselves might well take caution to be certain that their method of diagnosing TAB is correct before propounding their ideas about the relevance of this disorder to CHD. The possible errors inherent in epidemiological data recently have been pointed out by the epidemiologists themselves (Feinstein, 1988; Smith, Phillips, & Neaton, 1992), who point out the errors that may result when clinical acumen and plausibility are disregarded in the accumulation and statistical handling of sheer numbers.

My associates and I, intrigued by this statistical schism existing between the aforementioned investigators who found hostility the sole emotional precursor of CHD and those who did not, gave 21 of our postinfarction ambulatory participants in the Recent Coronary Prevention Project study

(Friedman et al., 1986) the same self-report employed by most of these investigators (i.e., the Cooke-Medley questionnaires). We also submitted these subjects to the videotaped clinical examination that is described in the next section. Twelve of the 21 participants given the questionnaires were found to report themselves as nonhostile. Twenty of the 21 participants, however, when given the videotaped clinical examination, were found to be not just hostile but severely so.

What does all this conflict concerning the positive or negative role hostility may play in the pathogenesis of CHD mean? I believe that all the investigators who employed some form of self-report for their diagnosis of hostility overlooked the verity that few persons are aware of their hostile ways and many of those who are aware of this unlovely TAB component are not anxious to reveal it. In short, whereas common sense may not be of much help in understanding quantum mechanics, it still plays a very important role in medicine.

INTRODUCTION OF THE VIDEOTAPED CLINICAL EXAMINATION FOR THE QUANTITATIVE DETECTION AND MEASUREMENT OF TAB

From the foregoing data, I believe that it is clear that a medical examination is an absolute prerequisite for the proper detection of the presence of TAB. This examination, which I have designated the videotaped clinical examination (VCE), attempts to elicit TAB symptoms and behavioral traits by employing a flexible enquiry by which the examiner learns about some of the basic features of the personality and behavior of the examinee, paying attention not only to the overt TAB components (time urgency and free-floating hostility) but also to the disorder's usual causal precursors of insecurity and/or inadequate self-esteem. Second, the examiner observes the examinee for his or her exhibition of those psychomotor signs indicative or suggestive of the presence of TAB.

For the detection of the time urgency and free-floating hostility components of TAB, three different groups of persons were subjected to this new diagnostic procedure. The findings then were submitted for biostatistical analyses.

Group 1 consisted of 99 male ambulatory postinfarction patients (average age, 54 years) randomly selected from 900 postinfarction subjects recruited in the Recurrent Coronary Prevention Project (Friedman et al.,

1986). Three of this group were Afro-American and the remainder were Caucasian. Most of the 99 patients were found to exhibit TAB when examined by an earlier similar diagnostic procedure that lacked, however, eight of the diagnostic manifestations that are utilized in the present examination, which will be described.

In reexamining the 99 of 900 postinfarction patients, we reasoned that for any diagnostic test to be considered valid, it should detect TAB in the overwhelming majority of known coronary patients. Expressed differently, since essentially all postinfarction subjects under 65 years were found to exhibit TAB by this earlier but less sophisticated examination (Friedman et al., 1986), any new diagnostic procedure that failed to detect more cases of TAB in these same coronary patients could not be considered an improved diagnostic instrument. In short, the 99 postinfarction subjects served as our "gold standard" TAB subjects.

Group 2 consisted of 23 subjects who were "gold standard" type B subjects. One subject was a male Afro-American and the remaining were male Caucasians. Their average age was 56 years. Except for several of these subjects, all men had been diagnosed as type B in 1960–1961 in the Western Collaborative Group Study (Rosenman et al., 1975) and again 17 years later when they served as controls in the Recurrent Coronary Prevention Project (Friedman et al., 1986). The several type B subjects who had not been diagnosed and followed for several or more decades were executives who had been observed for a number of years by three or more of their business associates. None had ever been observed to exhibit any episodes of either time urgency or free-floating hostility. None of the group had ever suffered any clinical manifestations of CHD. The electrocardiograms of all 23 subjects were normal.

To test the possible predictive validity of the new procedure, the total diagnostic scores of another group of 15 men (group 3) who were free of all clinical symptoms and electrocardiographic signs of CHD at the time of their examination, but who subsequently (2–12 months) developed symptoms and signs of clinical CHD, were collected and compared with the examination scores of groups 1 and 2 individuals. Seven of the men showed angiographic evidence of severe coronary artery obstructions. The remaining men suffered a documented myocardial infarction. Their average age was 56 years and all were Caucasian.

In this study employing the VCE, we (Friedman & Ghandour, 1993) searched for the 19 manifestations of time urgency (7 symptoms/traits and 12 psychomotor signs) and the 14 manifestations of free-floating hostility (7 symptoms/traits and 7 psychomotor signs). Each of the manifestations were given a numerical value (score). These scores were arbitrarily weighted to reflect the frequency of their presence in the gold standard 99 type A coronary patients and their rarity in the 23 gold standard type B subjects. For example, the TAB manifestation—chronic facial tension—which was observed in over half of the coronary patients but not in any of the type B subjects, was scored as 25. On the other hand, although another manifestation—hand clenching—was observed in the majority of coronary or group 1 patients, it also was observed in 8 of the 23 type B subjects of group 2. Consequently, its score was weighted as only 5.

For the detection of the presence of insecurity/inadequate self-esteem, two additional groups of men were recruited and subjected to the VCE to detect the possible presence of the two overt TAB components as well as the possible presence of TAB's covert component—insecurity/inadequate self-esteem—and to determine the possible correlation between the overt and covert components of the disorder.

Detection of the Manifestations of Time Urgency

I shall list below the manifestations indicative or suggestive of the presence of time urgency (impatience), the first of the two overt components of TAB. I also shall describe our own methods for discerning the not-always self-apparent presence of those physical or psychomotor signs associated with time urgency.

But a word of caution. Do not adhere too rigidly to my suggested methods of enquiry, regardless of the personality of the examinee encountered. To do so will mimic the fallible stereotype of a questionnaire or so-called "structured interview," not a truly medical search for the diagnostic symptoms and attributes of TAB. For example, if an examinee is a single person or has never driven a car, some of our suggested eliciting queries cannot be employed and the examiner must substitute a different question or mode of enquiry.

A description of the manifestations follows.

Elicitation of Symptoms and Traits of Time Urgency

1. Speed in walking, eating, and haste in leaving dinner table (5–15)[*]
   Eliciting queries: Do you walk fast (5); eat fast (5)? After you have eaten your dinner, do you like to continue sitting and chatting with members of your family or do you leave the table immediately (5)?

*Numerals in parentheses represent score values for calculating the total VCE score.

2. Advice by others to slow down (15)
   Eliciting query: Does your spouse or any intimate friend ever tell you to slow down, become less tense, or take it easier?
3. Intense dislike of waiting in lines (10)
   Eliciting query: Does it bother or upset you to wait in grocery checkout, banking, or theater lines or to be seated in a restaurant? (A vigorously expressed dislike is considered a scoring response.)
4. Involvement in polyphasic activities (5–15)
   Eliciting queries:
   a. Do you usually look at television or read a magazine or newspaper and also eat at the same time? (5)
   b. Do you examine your mail or do other things while listening to someone on the telephone? (5)
   c. Do you often think of other matters while listening to your spouse or others? (5)
5. Self-awareness of time urgency (20)
   Eliciting query: Do you believe that usually you are in a hurry to get things done?
6. Infrequent recall of memories, observation of natural phenomena, or daydreaming (10)
   Eliciting query: Do you frequently recall old memories, or just sit and daydream or meditate, or observe carefully flowers, trees, animals, or birds? (A scoring response is failure of examinee to do any of these things.)
7. Extreme punctuality (10)
   Eliciting query: If you make an appointment with someone, say at noon, will you be there? (A scoring response to this question is an intensely expressed, "I'm never late," or "I'd be there on the dot or even a few minutes before noon," or "I'd certainly be there and I'd be angry if the other person keeps me waiting." The type B person quite calmly responds, "Usually," or "I'd try to be there.")

Detection of TAB Psychomotor Signs of Time Urgency

The ability to detect the physical or psychomotor signs indicative or suggestive of the presence of either of the two overt components of TAB is not an easily learned faculty. It requires, indeed demands, as much training as a medical student expends in learning how to detect and identify heart murmurs, skin rashes, or abnormalities in the size or sensitivity of abdominal organs. Unfortunately, few psychologists have been trained, as have medical students, to employ their eyes and ears as diagnostic tools. As a consequence, it has been my experience that physicians usually become more quickly adept than psychologists in recognizing the often subtle but telltale physical signs indicative of the presence of TAB.

This does not mean that psychologists (and also psychiatrists) cannot become adept in detecting the psychomotor signs of TAB. Too often, however, they continue to believe that perhaps some sort of questionnaire can be found that alone may detect the presence of TAB. This deeply entrenched belief too often encourages such psychologists to avoid or delay the self-training of their ears and eyes to detect the psychomotor signs of this disorder. As we already emphasized, much of the confusion and controversy surrounding the role of TAB in the pathogenesis of CHD stems from this failure to detect the psychomotor signs that may provide the only indication of the presence of this medical disorder.

A description of the psychomotor signs suggestive or indicative of the time urgency component of TAB now follows:

1. Rapid speech (10)
   Examinee speaks at 140 or more words per minute, sometimes making it difficult to comprehend all that he says.
2. Tense posture—abrupt, rapid, jerky movements (5)
   Examinee sits tensely and/or his movements are hurried and abrupt.
3. Hastening speech of others (20)
   Examinee, when listening to others talking, frequently utters rapidly "uh huh, uh huh" or "mmh, mmh," to hasten unconsciously the rate of speech of others. The presence of only this one sign strongly suggests the presence of TAB.
4. Ticlike elevation of eyebrows (5)
   If present, it appears 3–10 times during the 15- to 20-minute examination period.
5. Ticlike elevation or retraction of one or both shoulders (5)
   It usually appears at similar frequency as sign 4.
6. Chronic facial tension (20)
   This sign requires considerable training, not necessarily to detect but to differentiate from facial hostility. It is due to tautness of the maxilla–masseter muscle complex, often accompanied by moderate contraction of the frontalis muscle. The eyelids frequently are narrowed.
7. Prolepsis (20)
   Three questions are asked of the examinee by the examiner after he or she first relates, in a tedious, pleonastic fashion, a mundane

circumstance that enhances the impatience of the examinee. Having done this, the examiner then slowly poses his/her question; however, before he or she finishes it, he or she begins to stutter. He or she notes whether the examinee, already aware of the end of this question, becomes proleptic. An example of such a presentation follows:

The examiner begins by saying, "Most working people usually arise before 8:00 AM during the weekdays." The examiner then purposely becomes pleonastic by adding, "That is, Monday through Friday. Of course, on Saturday and Sunday they may sleep later."

Having said this, the examiner then begins to ask the experimental question: "Now in your own case, Mr. James, during the weekdays, what time do you usually" . . . and then he or she begins to stutter, or stumble, saying "uh-uh-uh-uh."

The test is positive if the examinee interrupts the stumbling by himself or herself, finishing the question or answering the question before it is fully delivered. This questioning procedure is performed at least three times during the examination, employing a different question for each exercise. If the examinee interrupts and finishes the examiner's questioning sentences two out of three times, the result is considered a scoring response.

8. Tongue–teeth clicking (5–20)
   This clicking sound is created by the abrupt separation of the anterior part of the tongue from its prior adhesion to the back of the upper incisors, when the mouth is opened to speak. This tongue pressure against these upper teeth occurs reflexly when the maxilla–masseter muscle complex becomes tense. If this latter muscle tension becomes habitual and intense enough, then the tongue-to-teeth pressure becomes chronic, occasionally resulting in permanent indentations of the tongue (see Figs. 3.1 and 3.2).
   (NOTE: If just clicking is heard, the scoring response is 5; but if tongue disfiguration is observed, the score is 20.)

9. Audible, forced inspiration of air (10)
   The examinee is observed at times, especially when he or she is speaking rapidly, to suck in breaths of air as he or she continues to speak.

10. Expiratory sighs (5–20)
    Sometimes type B subjects emit an expiratory sigh, but if an examinee is observed to sigh more than once during the examination period, a score of 5 is given; if more than 5 times, a

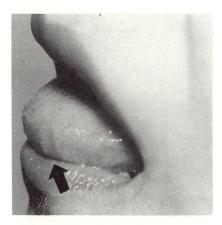

Figure 3.1. Arrow points to indentation of anterolateral portion of tongue of a young woman exhibiting severe type A behavior. Depressed area is due to chronic pressure of this area of the tongue against back of upper incisor tooth. (From Friedman & Ghandour, 1993. Reprinted with permission.)

score of 20 is given. It often is a sign of subliminal, emotional exhaustion.

11. Frequent eyelid blinking (5)

A scoring response is given if the examinee blinks 25 or more times per minute.

12. Excessive facial perspiration (40)

Chronic extrusion of beads of perspiration from the skin of the forehead and upper lip of the examinee or frequent daubing of the forehead with a handkerchief at normal room temperature. This is perhaps the most ominous of all TAB psychomotor signs, and if this is the only manifestation observed in an examinee, he or she must be diagnosed as suffering from severe TAB. We believe this excessive facial perspiration indicates an extreme, continuous discharge of the sympathetic nervous system.

In a sense, this sign is as prognostically portentous as the discovery of a neoplastic metastasis. We have observed that subjects exhibiting this sign invariably suffer some form of cardiovascular disaster before the age of 65 years.

[NOTE: Excessive perspiration in other parts of the body (e.g., axillae, hands or feet) is not necessarily of similar prognosis.]

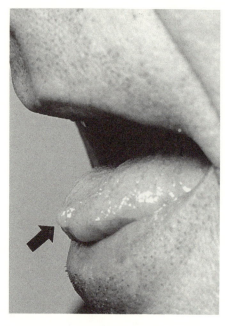

Figure 3.2. Arrow points to translucent benign growth at tip of tongue of a 48-year-old severely afflicted TAB man. He chronically pressed his tongue into a gap between two upper incisor teeth. (From Friedman & Ghandour, 1993. Reprinted with permission.)

Detection of the Manifestations of Free-Floating Hostility

The detection of free-floating hostility, the second overt component of TAB, is accomplished, as for the discovery of time urgency, through the elicitation of the symptoms/traits and the psychomotor signs indicative or suggestive of the presence of hostility or anger. A description of these manifestations follows.

Elicitation of Symptoms and Traits of Free-Floating Hostility

1. Sleeplessness because of anger/frustration (10)
    Eliciting query: Do you often find it difficult to fall asleep or difficult to stay asleep because you are upset about something a person has done? (A scoring response is one in which the examinee relates that the phenomenon is a common event.)

2. Disbelief in altruism (5)
   Eliciting query: Do you believe that most people are not honest or are not willing to help others? (A scoring response is an affirmative answer.)

3. Frequent loss of temper while driving (10)
   Eliciting queries: Do you become irritated when driving, especially while commuting? Does your spouse, when driving with you, ever tell you to cool or calm down? Do you swear at other drivers? (A scoring response is an affirmative answer to any of these questions.)

4. Marital tension or competition (15)
   Eliciting query: Do you have any feeling that your spouse is competing against you or is too critical of your inadequacies? (A scoring response is made if the examinee states that he or she has these feelings often or if his or her voice becomes bitter or his or her face becomes perturbed as he or she answers the questions.)

5. Teeth grinding (25)
   Eliciting query: Do you grind your teeth or has your dentist ever told you that you have done so?

6. Chronic difficulty in filial relationships (10)
   Eliciting query: Do you find (or have you found) it difficult dealing with your children? (Almost all parents may encounter some difficulties in dealing with their children, particularly when the latter are adolescent. The examiner, therefore, should not content himself or herself with asking a single question, but should ask a sufficient number to get a complete understanding of the present and past filial relationships of the examinee. Also, careful note should be made of the possible emergence of psychomotor signs in the examinee as he or she responds to this question. For example, if the voice of the examinee becomes strident or if his or her face clouds up as he or she discusses the question, a scoring response is indicated regardless of the content of his/her answers.)

7. Easily provoked irritability or discomfort on encountering the trivial errors of commission or omission by others (15)
   Eliciting query: Can you tell me what things annoy or upset you? [A quick answer by the examinee in which he or she lists, frequently in an unpleasant voice, several or more trivial matters (e.g., the car-driving errors of other drivers, the indifference of store clerks, or the tardiness of mail delivery) are scoring responses.]

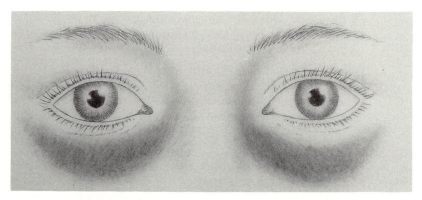

Figure 3.3. Shading of lower eyelid shows bilateral deposition of melaninlike pigment observed in varying degrees of intensity in approximately 27% of TAB persons. Pigmentation often involves upper eyelid and upper area of cheeks. (From Friedman & Ghandour, 1993. Reprinted with permission.)

Detection of Psychomotor Signs of Free-Floating Hostility

1. Periorbital pigmentation (25)
   A diffuse and permanent deposit of melanin, which imparts a brown color to the skin of the lower eyelid, although not infrequently a deposit also involves the upper eyelid (see Fig. 3.3). Its detection strongly suggests the presence of TAB regardless of whether other manifestations are elicited or detected.
2. Facial hostility (25)
   The physiognomy indicative of hostility is created by a combination of subtle but definite contractions of the orbital muscles, of the muscles surrounding the mouth, and of the masseter muscles. (For illustration and further information, see Fig. 3.4.)
3. Hostile laugh (10)
   Laughter that is jarring or explosive in character and often extraordinarily loud. In short, if the laugh appears unpleasant in pitch, tone, or volume to the examiner, a positive score is indicated.
4. Clenched hand in casual conversation (5–10)
   This physical sign, while frequently observed in coronary patients, is sometimes observed in healthy type B subjects. If the hand is

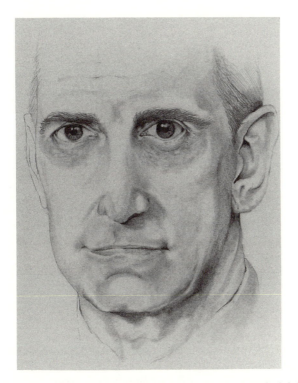

Figure 3.4. Hostility portrayed in this drawing is created by a combination of subtle but definite contractions of orbital muscles, muscles surrounding mouth, and masseter muscles. Glaring of eyes is created by retraction of upper eyelids through action of levator palpebrae muscles; this results in exposure of a larger portion of iris. In addition, lacrimal segment of orbicularis oculi muscles appears to raise the medial third of the lower lid slightly, thereby increasing intensity of stare. The corrugator portion of orbicularis oculi muscles lowers eyebrows to achieve further accentuation of perceived glare. Tightness or pursing of lips is achieved through tension in orbicularis oris muscle. Combined with bilateral pulling of risorius muscles, thinning of vermillion surface of lips occurs, and a "pseudosmile" appears. Glare of the eyes, "pseudosmile," and a slight bulge of tensed masseter muscles of jaw create a look of anger under a thin veneer of civility. A slight deposit of melanin is present on the lower eyelids. (From Friedman & Ghandour, 1993. Reprinted with permission.)

clenched and also pounded upon a desk or table, the scoring value should be increased from 5 to 10.

5. Ticlike bilateral retraction of the buccinator and orbicularis oris muscles (25)

A rapid, short retraction of the sides of the mouth sometimes sufficiently to expose the teeth (see Fig. 3.5).

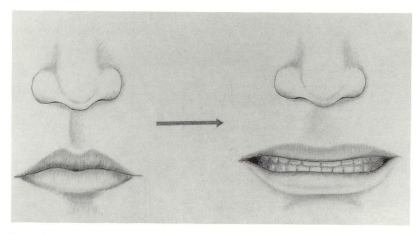

Figure 3.5. Sketch showing ticlike retraction of bilateral portions of the lips toward the ears (right), leading to partial opening of mouth often exposing distal ends of teeth. Sometimes retraction is extensive and may last several seconds. (From Friedman & Ghandour, 1993. Reprinted with permission.)

6. Ticlike retraction of upper (and sometimes lower) eyelid of either one or both eyes (25)
   A quick, abrupt, partial retraction of the upper eyelid (sometimes accompanied by a similar retraction of the lower eyelid) that briefly exposes the sclera above the iris (see Figs. 3.6 and 3.7).
7. Hostile voice (25)
   A speaking voice that is grating, harsh, irritating, excessively loud or just generally unpleasant, warrants a positive score.

The Detection of Insecurity/Inadequate Self-Esteem and Its Correlation with the Overt Components of TAB

There are eight queries in the VCE designed to detect the possible presence of insecurity/inadequate self-esteem (the covert TAB component). Two groups of previously ascertained type A subjects (191) and type B subjects (13) responded to these eight queries, as well as undergoing the remainder of the VCE for the detection of the two overt TAB components. The eight queries are:

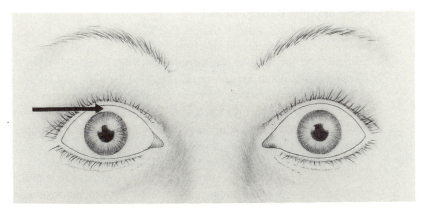

Figure 3.6. Sketch showing ticlike exposure of sclera above the iris (arrow indicates exposed sclera) caused by retraction of the upper eyelid. Sometimes the lower eyelid may also retract, exposing the sclera below the iris.

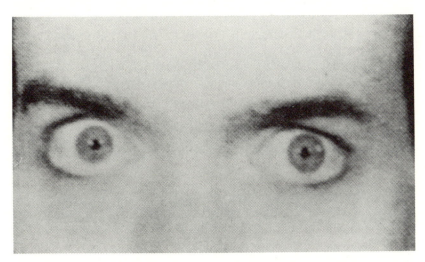

Figure 3.7. Photograph showing ticlike retraction of both the upper and lower eyelids of a TAB man. Note that the sclera is exposed both above and below the iris. (From Friedman & Ghandour, 1993. Reprinted with permission.)

1. Affection from other persons (5)
   Eliciting query: Do most of the people you know like you quite a bit? (A scoring response is an unequivocal "NO" reply.)
2. Sufficient or unconditional affection from both parents (15)
   Eliciting query: Most Type A people say that they did not receive sufficient or unconditional affection from both their parents. In your case, did you receive unconditional love and affection from both your parents? A scoring response is given if either parent did not give such affection.
3. Insecurities about finances, marriage, or career (5–10–20)
   Eliciting query: Do you, like most people, have insecurities about your finances, your marriage, or your career? A scoring response is 5 if examinee replies "sometimes," 10 if "often," and 20 if "constantly or too often."
4. Possible social inferiority (5–15)
   Eliciting query: On entering a room filled with your acquaintances or business associates, do you ever feel that too few of them wish to talk with you or sit next to you at a lunch or dinner table? A scoring response is 5 if response is "sometimes," and 15 if response is "very often."
5. Conversational inferiority (5–10)
   Eliciting query: In conversations with three or more persons, do you feel that they speak to each other more than to you? A scoring response is 5 if reply is "occasionally," and 10 if response is "frequently."
6. Attendance at your funeral or memorial service (5)
   Eliciting query: At your funeral or memorial service, do you believe a large number of persons will attend? A scoring response is 5 if reply is "No."
7. Difficulty in daydreaming or recalling memories (10)
   Eliciting query: Do you find it difficult to just sit and daydream or recall pleasant memories? A scoring response is 10 if reply is "Yes."
8. Covert feeling of failure (5–15–20)
   Eliciting query: William James wrote that if one finds the happiest man, the one most envied by the world, nine times out of ten his inmost consciousness is one of failure. Is this true in your case? A scoring response is 5 if reply is "yes, somewhat," 15 if reply is "Yes, that's how I frequently feel," and 20 if reply is "Yes, that's how I always feel."

Table 3.1. Correlation between Insecurity/Inadequate Self-Esteem and VCE

	Type A subjects	Type B subjects	Correlation coefficient[a]
Number of subjects	191	13	
Total VCE score	146	12	0.62 ($P < 0.0001$)
Time urgency score	96	7.6	0.57 ($P < 0.0001$)
Free-floating hostility	50	4.4	0.53 ($P < 0.0001$)
Insecurity/inadequate self-esteem	45	5.8	

[a]This is the coefficient correlation between insecurity/inadequate self-esteem scores and those of the total VCE, time urgency, and free-floating hostility scores of the total cohort.

As Table 3.1 demonstrates, the insecurity/inadequate self-esteem score of the type A subjects was eight times greater than that of the type B subjects. Table 3.1 also indicates that a strong correlation exists between the insecurity/inadequate self-esteem scores and those of the total VCE, as well as both its overt components.

The detection of the covert component is done solely by the elicitation of its possible symptoms and traits. But unlike the procedure for the detection of time urgency and free-floating hostility, we have not been able to observe any specific psychomotor sign specifically diagnostic of insecurity/inadequate self-esteem. Also, as we earlier have pointed out, insecurity/inadequate self-esteem may underlie and be responsible for an anxiety state or depression. Because of these reasons, for the diagnosis of TAB, we employ only the combined scores of time urgency and free-floating hostility, the TAB overt components.

The VCE Scores of the Three Groups

A profound difference was observed (see Table 3.2) between the average total VCE scores [i.e., the combined time urgency (TU) and free-floating hostility (FFH) scores] of the 99 coronary patients (group 1)

Table 3.2. Average Scores of VCE and Its Components in Coronary Patients and Type B Subjects

	Coronary patients[a] ($n = 99$)	Type B subjects ($n = 23$)
Time urgency component	78.1 (26.0)	15.5 (15.5)
Free-floating hostility component	23.3 (13.5)	0.7 (2.9)
Total VCE	101.4 (35.5)	16.3 (15.3)

[a]Figures in parentheses, standard deviation.

and the average total VCE score of the type B subjects (group 2). The total score of the former was 101.4 ($\pm$ 35.5) and that of the latter, 16.3 ($\pm$ 15.3). The average TU and FFH scores of the coronary patients were 78.1 ($\pm$ 26.0) and 23.3, respectively (see Table 3.2). The average total VCE scores of the 23 type B subjects was 16.3 ($\pm$ 15.83). The individual scores varied from 5 to 32. The average TU and FFH scores were 15.6 ($\pm$ 15.5) and 0.65 ($\pm$ 2.3), respectively (see Table 3.2).

The average total VCE scores of the group 3 participants who were examined prior to the onset of their clinical CHD was 133 (range, 38–207; SD, 50), a score greater (but not significantly so) than that (101.4) observed in the postinfarction subjects of group 1. Their average VCE score was significantly greater ($P < 0.001$) than that (16.3) observed in the type B subjects of group 2.

Almost three fourths of the total VCE score in group 1 postinfarction patients (see Table 3.2) and two thirds of the total VCE score in group 3 participants is contributed by the time urgency component. This is probably due to the fact that 19 of the 33 diagnostic type A manifestations are concerned with the presence of time urgency.

Prevalence of TU and FFH Manifestations in Group 1 Postinfarction Patients and Group 2 Type B Subjects

Each of the 99 group 1 postinfarction patients (see Table 3.3) possessed at least 5 of the 33 TU and FFH manifestations. The average number of manifestations was 11 per subject. Nine of the 11 manifestations were diagnostic of the presence of time urgency.

In striking contrast (see Table 3.3), 7 of the 23 group 2 type B subjects possessed none of the 33 manifestations. The average number of manifestations per subject was two. Here again, the manifestations were only diagnostic of the presence of TU.

Table 3.3. Average Number of TU and FFH Manifestations in Coronary Patients and Type B Subjects

	Average number of TU and FFH manifestations per subject	Average number of TU manifestations per subject	Average number of FFH manifestations per subject
Coronary patients ($n = 99$)	11.0 (5–18)	9.5 (5–15)	1.5 (0–5)
Type B subjects ($n = 23$)	2.5 (0–5)	1.8 (0–5)	0.65 (0–1)

Each of the group 3 subjects possessed at least 6 of the 33 TU and FFH manifestations. The average number of manifestations was 12 per subject. Similar to the group 1 subjects, the majority of manifestations observed in these subjects also were indicative of the presence of TU.

In summary, the group 3 subjects possessed and exhibited the same number and kind of manifestations prior to their suffering from clinical CHD as did those who were examined after their clinical CHD had occurred.

Determination of the Optimal Diagnostic Cutoff Score Values of the Total VCE and Its Components' Scores

The truly helpful type A diagnostic process will be one that will be most sensitive, specific, and efficient in detecting a coronary patient or coronary-prone subject and differentiating such persons from those who are relatively immune to clinical CHD (i.e., type B subjects). With this goal in mind and employing the score values obtained from our examinations of groups 1 and 2, the biometrician of our project, Ghassan Ghandour, employed the receiver operating characteristic (ROC) methodology (McNeel, Keller, & Adelstein, 1975; Swets & Pichett, 1982) to determine which of the cutoff values of the three scores (total, TU, FFH) would provide the greatest diagnostic:

1. Sensitivity: The proportion of postinfarction subjects identified correctly as type A.
2. Specificity: The proportion of type B subjects identified correctly as type B.
3. Efficiency: The proportion of the total group of both types A and B individuals correctly identified.

Dr. Ghandour concluded after his statistical analyses of groups 1 and 2 that total VCE cutoff scores of 45 or above detected and differentiated the coronary patients of group 1 from the type B subjects of group 2. Employing this cutoff score value, 97 of the 99 coronary patients (98%) of group 1 but only 1 of the 23 type B men were diagnosed as type A.

The optimal cutoff score, if only TU manifestations were employed for diagnosing TAB, was found to be 43. The optimal cutoff score, if only the FFH manifestations were employed, was found to be 5. However, if the cutoff score of just the TU manifestations was employed, 9 of the 99 coronary patients would have been diagnosed as type B and, conversely, 2 of the 23 type B subjects would have been diagnosed as type A subjects. Moreover, if only the TU manifestations of symptoms and traits were searched for and scored, but the TU psychomotor signs were overlooked, 17 of the 99 coronary patients would have been diagnosed as possessing type B behavior.

Employment of the optimal cutoff score, 5, obtained from the detection and scoring of only the FFH manifestations proved even more fallible. Thus, 18 of the 99 coronary patients (18%) would have been diagnosed as type B. If the optimal cutoff score of just the FFH symptoms and traits was employed, 44 of the 99 coronary patients (44%) would be diagnosed as type B subjects.

It is obvious from these results that the total VCE (i.e., the sum of both the TU and FFH manifestations) is superior to either single component in detecting and differentiating type A coronary patients from healthy type B subjects Also, as Table 3.1 demonstrates, using the cutoff total VCE score of 45 proves the most sensitive, specific, and efficient diagnostic process.

A VCE score value of 45 or one considerably higher, of course, does not indicate that the subject harbors clinical CHD or ever will. However, it has been our experience, with no remembered exception, that a person exhibiting a total VCE score below 45 not only does not possess clinical CHD, he will remain immune to its onset well past his 60th birthday.

Single Warning Signs of TAB

We have listed in the preceding paragraphs the overt manifestations by which TAB can be diagnosed and its intensity quantitatively assessed. The VCE also permits the detection of the underlying insecurity/inadequate self-esteem almost always present in the behavioral disorder.

However, certain of the previously listed manifestations are almost always diagnostic of the presence of TAB even if it is the only manifestation elicited or observed. They are the following:

1. Self-awareness and admission of the presence of impatience or easily induced hostility.
2. Teeth grinding.
3. Prolepsis.
4. Excess perspiration of the forehead and the upper lip.
5. Indentation of the tongue due to its chronic pressure against the upper incisor teeth.
6. Ticlike retraction of the upper eyelid.

Table 3.4.   Comparison of TAB Manifestations in TAB Men and
Women

	TAB men	TAB women
Number	2758	272
Total VCE score	169	176
Time urgency score	108	117
Free-floating hostility score	61	59
Insecurity/inadequate self-esteem	51	57[a]

[a]Significantly greater (p < 0.0003) than analogous score of TAB men.

7. Ticlike retraction of the lateral corners of the mouth.
8. Periorbital pigmentation.

The Diagnostic Manifestations of TAB in Women

The diagnostic manifestations of time urgency, hostility, and insecurity/inadequate self-esteem in 272 TAB women were compared with analogous manifestations in 2758 TAB men. All of the individuals were 45 years or older, were ostensibly free of CHD, and had volunteered to participate in our ongoing Coronary/Cancer Prevention Project.

As Table 3.4 illustrates, not only was the total VCE score essentially the same in the two groups, but the scores of time urgency and free-floating hostility were also approximately the same. The degree of insecurity/inadequate self-esteem in the TAB women was significantly greater than that observed in the TAB men. It thus seems certain that the diagnostic manifestations of the overt components of TAB are essentially the same in both sexes. Not surprisingly, the TAB woman apparently harbors a greater sense of insecurity/inadequate self-esteem.

II

Modification of Type A
Behavior

Qualities of an Effective Group Leader in Type A Counseling

I have had 19 years of experience in the selection of dozens of group leaders and subsequent observation of their effectiveness in modifying TAB. From this experience, it has been possible to observe the qualities possessed by those persons who achieved the greatest modification of TAB in the participants of their groups. These qualities are described below.

POSSESSION OF WISDOM

A large part of type A group counseling consists of encouraging the acquisition of wisdom in the group participants. This means that the group leader must possess this virtue.

It is not easy to define the sort of wisdom needed for successful type A counseling, although it is easy enough to define what is not wisdom. For example, the acquisition of academic knowledge or degrees is not necessarily commensurate with wisdom, nor is sheer intellectual brilliance. But the capacity to view objects and events in their true relationship or relative importance is a major component of wisdom; so are foresight and the valuable gift of insight. When all of these components are in proper balance in an individual, it may be designated as common sense. And common sense is not a commonly seen quality in the TAB person.

INTEGRITY OF CHARACTER

A group leader either does or does not possess integrity. If he or she does not, no one will discover this more rapidly than a group of TAB persons. As we have already pointed out, cynicism is a quality in such persons, and it is this quality that makes them unusually efficient in detecting character flaws in other people. Accordingly, once a group leader is even suspected of lacking integrity, his or her usefulness as a type A group leader ceases.

CAPACITY TO CARE FOR AND FEEL AFFECTION FOR GROUP PARTICIPANTS

A group participant receiving type A counseling very quickly discerns whether his or her group leader cares for him or her or whether he or she is viewed impersonally as just one of the 15 other group participants who are completely forgotten by the group leader once any given session ends. Because too often the type A person has unconsciously been yearning for the love and affection he or she should have but did not receive as a youngster, he or she would like to believe that the group leader is able to care for him or her as an individual. If he or she does not receive such attention, he or she loses faith very quickly in the group leader, and the latter's possible effectiveness in modifying the participant's TAB is almost nil.

TOTAL ABSENCE OF THE HOSTILITY AND CONSCIOUS CONTROL OF THE TIME URGENCY COMPONENT OF TAB

Obviously, a group leader who suffers from the free-floating hostility component of TAB cannot be expected to modify the intensity of this same component in his or her group participants. This is particularly the case because a group leader must teach his or her participants from the outset of their course how to detect the presence of this component in other persons.

On the other hand, a group leader can possess a moderate degree of time urgency. But the group leader must be able to keep it within the limits of simple urgency and not allow it to develop in outright impatience. Most importantly, the group leader should admit to his or her group participants that he or she does suffer to some degree a sense of time urgency at times, but that he or she usually is aware of and can soften the intensity of this TAB component.

POSSESSION OF A GOOD TO EXCELLENT BACKGROUND IN THE HUMANITIES

A good leader is expected to encourage his or her group participants to engage more of their time in "right-brain" activities (e.g., the appreciation of literature, painting, sculpture, and music), but he or she must be interested and knowledgeable to some extent in one or more of these activities. In a sense, the group leader's degree of wisdom is determined in part by his or her awareness of the value of the humanities.

SKILL IN ENGENDERING ENTHUSIASM IN GROUP PARTICIPANTS

Simply, to engender enthusiasm, the group leader must feel enthusiastic in doing his or her job and be able to display it to the group.

ABILITY TO MAINTAIN GROUP DECORUM

From the beginning, the group leader must exhibit the facial and vocal tones of decision and determination that comprise the charisma of leadership, as he or she will need determination in the control of his or her 15 group participants.

Second, the group leader must repeatedly insist that the group participants regularly perform their exercises and strengthen their self-criticizing monitor by its frequent use.

Third, the group leader frequently must remind the group participants to always keep in mind the changes in behavior that they initially desired to change. This is necessary because participants will only change their behaviors if they keep in mind the *specific* changes they initially wished to change.

Fourth, the group leader must see to it that although group discussions are to be encouraged, he or she must have the courage to interrupt and stop any pleonastic tendencies of individual participants. If this is not accomplished, the other participants eventually become bored or irritated with such performances, particularly if only one or two participants regularly indulge in this distraction.

Finally, the group leader must have the ability in all group discussions to see to it that these discussions focus only on those matters that affect or are affected by the overt and covert TAB components.

Presently, the Friedman Institute employs 23 group leaders in its ongoing research project in which 1500 individuals are receiving type A modification. Seventeen of these group leaders are psychologists, most of whom have received their doctorate in psychology. Two of the 23 group leaders are educators who received their doctorate in education. The remaining four group leaders are two internists and two psychiatrists. Eight of the 17 psychologists are female. All eight women possess the qualities I have listed. I believe that as group leaders they generally exhibit more care for their group participants than the male group leaders. Deprived as the majority of our type A participants were of unconditional love in their early youth, they particularly are positively affected by the sometimes sisterlike preoccupation of the female group leader. Certainly, as judged by repeat videotaped clinical examinations done 1–3 years after the entrance of type A persons into a modification course led by a woman, their degree of modification of the intensity of their TAB is as good as or even superior to that shown by those instructed by a male group leader.

5

Enhancement of Self-Esteem

As we earlier emphasized in describing insecurity/inadequate self-esteem, this covert and causative component for the emergence and continuation of the overt components of TAB pattern appears in the majority of cases to arise in early childhood because of insufficient display of affection and admiration from both parents. In such cases, free-floating hostility also appears before such children reach the age of 10. In most of the remaining cases, insecurity/inadequate self-esteem begins some time before or during adolescence. In these latter cases, insufficient parental affection and admiration do not appear to have triggered the onset of this emotional perturbation.

SELF-DETECTION BY TAB SUBJECTS OF THEIR INADEQUATE SELF-ESTEEM AND INSECURITY

Because of its salient role in the pathogenesis of TAB, insecurity/inadequate self-esteem at onset should receive the attention of the group leader. However, because of its covert nature, many TAB subjects are not consciously aware of this component, or in other cases are reluctant to admit its presence. In view of these circumstances, the leader initially should approach the revelation and improvement of this covert component with some degree of caution and finesse, until the participant becomes comfortable with and accepting of the help given to him or her not only by the group leader but also by his or her fellow group participants.

We have found that the first measure to take is to distribute a small piece of blank paper at the first or second group session and

9

request that each participant respond with a "yes" or "no" answer to the following question: Did you receive sufficient affection and admiration from *both* your parents? Prior to their writing down their responses, it is explained that if they have been brought up by only one parent, their answer should be "no." They are also told not to sign their name on the paper but to fold it and hand it to the leader. The leader then hands all the folded paper responses to one of the participants and asks the participant to read off the responses, which the leader then tabulates on a blackboard or flip chart. Prior to tabulation, the group leader writes the numbers 60–90 in one corner. After all the "yes" and "no" responses are displayed, the group leader determines the percentage of "no" responses. Almost invariably this percentage will turn out to be over 60% regardless of whether the group is composed of type A men or women.

After demonstrating this calculation, the group leader then will point to the 60–90 number and declare that he or she knew from previous experiences with earlier groups that their "no" responses also would be more than 60%. He or she then emphasizes that for a subject to have scientific validity, it must possess predictability. The group leader resorts to this device because at the early stages of counseling, he or she has the task of convincing some of the participants who still remain skeptical of the scientific validity of the TAB concept and its possible relevance to their own disorder.

Immediately following the demonstration of this percentage of "no" responses, most group participants are shocked by the commonness of this parental aberration. They also feel less alone and somewhat relieved that all or most of their group members have experienced the same emotional deficit. Perhaps it is this demonstration that serves as the initial process of "bonding" the participants to one another.

This exposure of a common earlier misfortune makes it easier for group participants to discuss the individual aspects of their parental experiences in subsequent sessions. This procedure also encourages those few group members who did receive unconditional love from their parents to describe freely and in detail extraparental episodes that gave rise to the beginning of their insecurity/inadequate self-esteem. Certainly, within the first six group sessions, the TAB participants not only become aware of their insecurity/inadequate self-esteem and its causes, but they also feel free in discussing these causes and their possible remedies with their group leader and their fellow participants.

SUBSTITUTION OF NEW FOR OLD BELIEF SYSTEMS

NEW BELIEF: *The things worth being deserve as much attention or, in many cases, even more than that given to the things worth having*

This particular belief represents more a philosophical than a purely psychological belief, but it bears directly on what we already have emphasized: the failure of the accumulation of merely material things or even power to remedy insecurity/inadequate self-esteem. Certainly, if accumulation alone increasingly preoccupies the personality, then the intellectual and spiritual interest and curiosity of this same personality in the arts, music, and literature as well as the joy in persons, pets, and plants—the "things worth being"—receives a devastating blow (even if it has not been self-perceived).

But the loss of the "things worth being" is not always caused by the acquisition of material objects. Darwin (cited in James, 1890), for example, observed his growing distaste for poetry, music, and the arts, which he believed was a sign of "atrophy of that part of the brain on which alone higher tastes depend (p. 446)." He further believed that this atrophy was caused by his mind becoming "a kind of machine for grinding general laws out of large collections of facts (p. 446)." Darwin confessed that he did not know how this use of his mind did away with some of the "things worth being" in his later life.

Roger Sperry, however, who won the Nobel prize in 1981 for discovering the predominance of the left hemisphere over the "silent" right cerebral hemisphere, could have given Darwin at least part of the answer. He would have explained to Darwin that the left brain flourishes on its increasing input and output of numbers and sheer facts. Such development functionally suppresses the right brain, where matters of music, poetry, art, and vivid imagination struggle just to exist, much less flourish.

In general, type A women, unlike most type A men, already realize that the things worth being more often than not exceed the things worth having. Their spouses, however, being type A, too often presuppose that they can be satisfied with the possession of material things.

NEW BELIEF: *The emotional deprivation experienced in childhood by the majority of TAB participants cannot be alleviated by the sole accumulation of things and power*

It is unfortunate that the majority of type A participants who are not given sufficient parental affection and admiration, in seeking compensation for this unfilled need, usually do not seek to find these spiritually nourishing components from persons other than their parents. Rather, they strive to acquire things and achieve power and dominance over their colleagues. Their intent, which intensifies as they grow older, is an often unconscious desire to acquire and dominate even at the cost of the envy and hatred of their contemporaries.

The acquisition of things and power over other persons, however, does not enhance the security or self-esteem of the TAB participant. It seems at best an ephemeral palliative that ends in worsening, not improving, self-esteem.

The first step to be taken by the TAB participant to diminish his or her long-suffered childhood injury is to forgive his or her mother or father for their failures to give him or her the love he or she needed and to find ways to feel compassion for their perhaps unpreventable errors. The TAB participant, whether woman or man, must be encouraged frequently to remember and accept the truth of this fact: No one ever diminished his or her self-esteem by forgiving another for his/her mistakes.

NEW BELIEF: *Frequent recall of certain past achievements and episodes of happiness can enhance one's self-esteem*

Whatever confidence a champion athlete—whether a boxer, golfer, tennis player, or pole vaulter—possesses as he or she enters into a new contest stems from the memory of victories enjoyed in the past. This truth is easily understood if one considers how this same champion might feel if, on the morning of a new contest, he or she awakened with a complete loss of memory. In a not so limited sense, this is precisely from what so many TAB participants suffer. They habitually become so preoccupied with possible future contingencies in which they may fail that they find little time or desire for a regular recollection of their past successes. Thus, no matter how great a prior accomplishment is in the career of a TAB person, a far less, often trivial, pending task or transaction raises the specter not just of its failure but far worse—the beginning of collapse of his or her entire career.

If a vocational career can be likened to a triangle whose base is composed of remembered past successes and accomplishments and whose apex is composed of new or future enterprises, the type B person, always consciously remembering his or her past achievements, knows that whatever in the future may damage the apex of his or her triangle, its intact base will prevent its toppling. Not so with the TAB subject. His or her triangle rests on its apex composed of future enterprises. It is his or her constant fear that if one such enterprise fails, its damage to the apex of his or her triangle will cause its total collapse.

A good example of this continuing fear of a future mishap leading to the total collapse of a career is the fear felt by ex-President Lyndon B. Johnson when there was a slight delay in the receipt of mechanical parts for the irrigation pumps of his ranch. Despite his total success as a senator, his partial successes as the president, and his totally secure multimillion dollar investments, Doris Kearns (1976) describes in her book his verbalized despair at the delay of pump parts: "It's all been determined, you know. Once more I am going to fail. I know it. All my life I've wanted to enjoy this land. It's all I have left now." Then the next morning Johnson complained to Ms. Kearns, "I couldn't sleep all night. Not a minute. I kept thinking about those pump parts. I must have those parts before the end of the day. I simply must. If I don't, everything's going to fall apart. Everything." The pump parts arrived several days later, giving Johnson relief of his anxiety about this particular minor mishap. Of course, Ms. Kearns reports a series of similar "crises" that occurred during her short stay with the ex-President at his Texas ranch.

On the other hand, the regular recall of past pleasant and happy incidents strengthens one's esteem. We visit new places or countries to enjoy their customs, scenery, historical landmarks, and so forth. But we would not bother to make such trips if we thought we would never remember later the experiences we encountered. Except too often the TAB person never finds times for such recall. He or she has forgotten what Emily Dickinson once wrote over a century ago: "Such good things can happen to people who learn to remember (p. 189)."

NEW BELIEF: *The sincere bestowal upon and the joyful acceptance of unconditional affection and admiration from one's spouse, children, and several or more friends serves as a powerful restorative of self-esteem*

Repeatedly, we have heard TAB group participants, after only a few months of counseling, declare: "I've got lots of acquaintances but no real friends." These same individuals also discover that, although they may even do favors for scores of their acquaintances, they find it exceedingly difficult or even impossible to maintain an ongoing, absorbing interest in the concerns and activities of these same acquaintances. The TAB man or woman may lunch with an acquaintance regularly and consider him or her a friend, but at the end of the lunch this friend and his or her interests, hopes, and activities disappear from the TAB person's consciousness until perhaps the next luncheon at which time the same emotional sort of dumb show will ensue.

Perhaps the first step for a TAB subject to take in establishing a meaningful friendship is to verbalize to potential friends the true regard he feels for his or her friend. For example, if a TAB person believes that a certain person is his or her best friend, he or she might tell him or her, "You are my best friend," or "I really look forward to our meetings."

But the next step, and it is the crucial one, is for the TAB participant to regularly remember some of the interests and ongoing activities of one or several of his or her friends in the interludes between their meetings. This interest in the lives, activities, and expectations of these friends should continue until such interest becomes a moderately absorbing avocation for the TAB person. Certainly the security and self-esteem of any individual never is threatened by his or her increased interest, affection, and admiration for one or more of his or her friends. A resurgence of expressed (i.e., verbal and physical) affection toward one's spouse and children also will not engender a deterioration in one's security or self-esteem.

I have found that unlike many type A men, type A women find it much easier to adopt this particular "new" belief of giving unconditional love and affection to members of her family and friends.

CONSTRUCTION OF A SELF-MONITOR

There is probably no more effective tool in enhancing the security or self-esteem of the TAB person than his or her construction of a monitor that vigilantly and immediately detects and modifies or abolishes any action or reaction of the TAB individual that might further increase his or her insecurity or inadequate self-esteem. For example, one of our participants, a president of a bank, when at a cocktail party or similar sort of social gathering that was often attended by the president of a bigger bank than his own invariably counted the number of guests who approached him and the number who approached the rival president. Because the number who approached the other president invariably exceeded the number who came to him, his self-esteem sank. After several months of group counseling, our participant's self-monitor upon spotting the other bank president at a party almost instantaneously "forbade" him to revert to his usual counting procedure. As a substitute, his self-monitor encouraged him to observe that those persons who did gravitate to him were far more his friends than those who clustered around the other president.

Also, as the self-monitor progressively develops, it almost instantaneously can stop the TAB participant from feeling or verbalizing cynical eruptions. Instead, it encourages him or her to remember that cynicism per se never increases self-esteem and often further erodes it.

The group leader plays the principal role in hastening the transition of the monitor from simple self-talk to a third person sort of guiding entity. He or she accomplishes this transformation by always emphasizing the word "monitor" in lieu of self-admonition. Thus, he or she asks, "What did your monitor advise you to do to rouse yourself from depression?" or "Why didn't your monitor prevent you from becoming fearful of embarking on that prospect?" Also, the leader at each session regularly asks different participants of his or her group how many times their monitor cautioned or advised them during the past 24 hours.

By repetitiously referring to the monitor as a distinct almost lifelike entity, the leader manages to effect its independence and its power to influence the emotional actions and reactions of its possessor. This evolution of previous, often ineffective, self-talk to a powerful, impersonal, unassailable (friendly) critic and advisor is a subtle one, often taking months to bring about. But its development and employment repeatedly have been credited by our TAB participants for the rapid diminution in their insecurity and enhancement of their self-esteem.

DAILY PERFORMANCE OF NEW HABIT-FORMING EXERCISES

I (Friedman & Ulmer, 1984) have found that certain habits that promote insecurity and inadequate self-esteem must be replaced with new and healthier ones. But these new habits are not easy to plant and take the place of various old ones. For this reason, involvement in exercises (or drills) aimed at enhancing the security and self-esteem of the group participants should be started at the beginning of the modification course.

Appendix 1 lists the 45 exercises or drills that we employed in modifying TAB in 2800 men during the past 15 years. As shown in the appendix, I have grouped these exercises in three categories according to their purpose and goal. Fifteen of these 45 exercises are designed to enhance security and self-esteem. The remaining are designed to alleviate time urgency/impatience and free-floating hostility and will be discussed in the subsequent two chapters. In short, from the beginning, just as the group participants are encouraged to change some of their belief systems, they concomitantly begin to perform these exercises.

Each participant receives a 24-page booklet corresponding to the 24 months of the 2-year course for modifying TAB. Each page contains seven exercises designed to enhance security/self-esteem or modify time urgency or free-floating hostility. The participant is to perform a different drill each day of the first week (see Appendix 2) and then the same drills are performed each day for the remaining 3 weeks of the first month.

Thus, group participants from the beginning perform exercises to alter both the covert (i.e., the insecurity/inadequate self-esteem) and the overt components (time urgency/impatience and free-floating hostility) of the TAB pattern. In Appendix 3, we have listed a number of suggestions that we have found helpful in our initial presentation of the exercises.

The group participants are instructed to write an "X" in the square enclosing each printed exercise. If the participants follow the leader's instructions, at the end of any month, each of the seven squares should exhibit four "Xs." Certainly, the exercise booklets should be inspected frequently by the group leader to make sure that his or her participants are performing their exercises.

DAILY CONTEMPLATION OF GENERAL TRUTHS AND PRINCIPLES OF CONDUCT

In addition to the seven general exercises to be done each week, we have printed on each of the 24 monthly pages of the booklet 4 of the 96 philosophically oriented quotations and maxims derived from various literary sources. Group participants are instructed to read and thoughtfully consider daily during the first week the first of the four quotations/maxims. Then, they continue to consider daily each of the remaining quotations/maxims for the second, third, and fourth weeks successively of each month. These 96 quotations/maxims are listed in Appendix 4.

This particular procedure does not influence the thinking and conduct of all participants equally. But repeatedly we have been impressed by the power that a single, particular one of these concepts can exert on the belief systems of various group participants.

Often, too, participants wish to discuss one of the quotations/maxims during a group session. Also, many of these quotations furnish the group leader the means of introducing subjects for group discussion. For example, discussion of Carl Jung's statement (see quotation 7 in Appendix 4), "No psychic value can disappear without being replaced by another of equal intensity," fortifies the group leader in his or her attempts to encourage the participants to substitute new beliefs for their old beliefs.

Again, Locke's quotation (see quotation 18 in Appendix 4), "One's personal identity is a chain of particular memories," serves as a powerful tool for the group leader to attempt to induce participants to regularly recall their past significant achievements for the enhancement of their self-esteem. This is because quoting Locke affords the leader the authority of a distinguished author whom the participants cannot help respecting and possibly paying heed to—a result that might not occur if the group leader had uttered the same statement but without attributing it to Locke.

Modification of Time Urgency and Impatience

Before meaningful diminution in the intensity of time urgency (and impatience) can be accomplished, individuals possessing the type A component of time urgency and impatience must first become cognizant of harboring it. After such recognition, they then must identify the underlying causes responsible for their time urgency. They then will be able to attempt to alter those belief systems that have sustained or aggravated this type A component. After such alteration, they must involve themselves in various specific exercises, or drills, to diminish the intensity of their sense of time urgency.

SELF-DETECTION BY TAB SUBJECTS OF THEIR TIME URGENCY

Although a major fraction of TAB subjects suffering from time urgency are unaware that they harbor this trait, when they receive even superficial instruction in identification of the symptoms, traits, and particularly the psychomotor signs of this TAB component, they are able to recognize quite rapidly its presence. These manifestations are described in Chapter 3.

SELF-RECOGNITION BY TAB SUBJECTS OF THE SPECIFIC CAUSE OF THEIR TIME URGENCY

The various causes that are responsible for the emergence and continuance of time urgency are listed and described in Chapters 1–3. As already stressed, a covert sense of insecurity or inadequate self-esteem underlies this type A component in almost all cases, but it is important for good therapeutic results to discover what other additional causes may be at play in each afflicted individual. For example, one person may intensify his or her sense of time urgency if he or she is unable to delegate tasks to subordinates, and thus finds insufficient time to accomplish all the enterprises that he or she has assumed, whereas another person may intensify sense of time urgency by his/her excessive pride in doing far more things than most other people can do in a given amount of time.

SUBSTITUTION OF NEW FOR OLD BELIEF SYSTEMS

NEW BELIEF: *Time urgency hinders, never enhances, a vocational career*

Unfortunately, the majority of male citizens in American urban communities, whether they be janitors or chief executive officers of major corporations, exhibit varying degrees of time urgency.* Given the relative ubiquity of this trait, it is easy to understand why so many individuals make the error of attributing whatever successes they have achieved in their industrial, commercial, or professional career to those actions of theirs that sustained or enhanced their time urgency.

It is therefore of prime importance to encourage persons afflicted with a sense of time urgency to recognize that their successes were due to such entities as:

1. Creative abilities.
2. Talent for efficient organization and systematization.
3. Capacity to execute often dull and tedious activities to attain desired goals.
4. Ability to gain the respect, admiration, and even affection of their subordinates, peers, and superiors.
5. Good fortune.

New participants, particularly type A women who have taken on executive positions in large corporations, often will cling to their mistaken belief that somehow or other time urgency and, yes, even impatience have

---

*An exception to this generalization may be embalmers. In recruiting type A and type B subjects in 1959, we found (Friedman & Rosenman, 1974) that most of these professional technicians did not suffer from time urgency. As the poet Emily Dickinson wrote of death, "He knew no haste."

been essential factors in those successes they have achieved. To combat this persistent belief, we have found it helpful to reduce type A behavior to its basic factors:

> A: Anger
> I: Irritability
> A: Aggravation
> I: Impatience

I then ask group participants if they really believe they can discover wonderful, creative ideas and contemplate their application while they harbor AIAI? Their answer invariably is "no."

NEW BELIEF: *Daily prioritization of one's activities*

There may be a number of persons who are not threatened with temporal inundation by the number of activities that confront them daily, but we do not believe that they constitute the major portion of any Western urban population. TAB persons are particularly susceptible to the pressure engendered by their feeling that there is not sufficient time to accomplish all the things that they believe they should accomplish. Moreover, this feeling is not helped by their tendency to delay performing tasks that are important but are tedious or dull (e.g., collecting data for one's income tax, filling out forms of various kinds, making out reports, etc.) Thus, their execution is delayed as far more trivial tasks are tackled.

Accordingly, TAB persons must be strongly and repeatedly urged to plan each day to tackle the most important (not necessarily those that appears pressing) problems, regardless of how tiresome or even irritating they may be. He or she must take care, as a lieutenant colonel of the War College taking our course in 1984 learned, not to expend ten dollars worth of effort on a ten cent activity.

NEW BELIEF: *Making time one's friend*

Most TAB persons feel that they are fighting time in that time appears habitually opposed to their efforts to accomplish all that they wish accomplished in any given day, week, or month. For these individuals, the deadline represents the basic hostility of time.

To make time one's friend, one must first remember that if no events took place, time as an entity would no longer exist. So it is the person and only the person who fashions the contour and consistency of time. If one would wish to transform time into a friendly and relatively flexible entity in one's life, one must cease assuming that time is some sort of infinitely extensible container into which one can unceasingly push more and more events.

If time is to become one's friend, one must stop struggling to achieve too many things in too little time. The first and best way of reaching this goal is to examine very carefully the temporal importance of one's activities. For example, any activity or event that does not have importance over a 5-year period may, more often than not, be dispensable. Such events are to be suspected and possibly censored if they produce deadlines, because a deadline automatically construes time as an enemy, never a friend. In short, the steps toward making a friend of time can be gauged by the increasing rarity of self-imposed, unnecessary, and often quite trivial deadlines.

NEW BELIEF: *It is never too late to diminish time urgency*

Because it is not easy to forego habits of haste of many years' duration, it is not uncommon for TAB subjects to avoid altering such habits by assuming that they are too old to attempt their modification. This is a belief that can only be countered effectively by the demonstration that it is a false one. I have found that the most effective measure to accomplish this is the exercise that alters long-established actions and reactions occurring during the driving of an automobile. This particular exercise will be described later in this chapter.

NEW BELIEF: *Let the means justify the end*

The TAB person, because of his or her covert insecurity, is so preoccupied with what might happen in the future and tries so often to forestall feared mishaps that he or she has neither the time nor the inclination to enjoy the present. This neglect subverts whatever joys and triumphs that a day's activities can provide so that, when not keenly appreciated, these activities totally fade into an irretrievable past. The type A subject excuses this neglect of the day's activities and events by rationalizing that his or her end justifies this sloughing away of his or her means.

This old belief in which the type A person loses both the present and past must be superseded by a new belief: The means justify the end. Such a change in beliefs can only evolve if the type A subject faces up to what his or her end really is: his or her death. Once convinced of the true nature of his or her end, he or she will not find it too difficult not only to appreciate the singular events of any given day but also to mark it so that it may be suitably recorded in his or her memory and easily recallable.

CONSTRUCTION OF A SELF-MONITOR

The self-monitor, described in Chapter 5, is probably the most effective of all tools in alleviating the intensity of time urgency. As in enhancing self-esteem, the self-monitor does not become fully effective in correcting or preventing time urgency until it becomes adept in (1) detecting all the psychomotor signs as well as the symptoms/traits of time urgency, (2) discovering the immediate causes for the acute eruption of this TAB component, and (3) obtaining complete and instantaneous obeisance in eliminating the immediate causes. The effectiveness of a monitor in preventing or bringing to a quick end an episode of time urgency is brought to light when subjects afflicted with time urgency make statements such as: "I was just about ready to get impatient but my monitor prevented it," or "My monitor stopped me from interrupting my friend's conversation so I just sat there and listened calmly to what he had to say."

DAILY PERFORMANCE OF NEW HABIT-FORMING EXERCISES

As we already discussed in Chapter 5, the elimination of old habits that engender and sustain the occurrence of time urgency/impatience requires their replacement with healthier habits that do not induce this overt TAB component.

The exercises or drills that are to be followed in order to modify the intensity of time urgency/impatience are listed in Appendix 1. These exercises form a fraction of the exercises that, together with those designed to enhance security/self-esteem and reduce free-floating hostility, compose the seven different exercises that make up the weekly regimen of drills (see Appendix 2) already described in Chapter 5.

Again, the group leader should regularly examine the exercise booklets of his or her participants to make sure that they are performing their daily drills. He/she also should enquire about their daily contemplation of one of the four maxims printed on each month's page (see Appendix 2).

A Special Exercise: Modification of Time Urgency and Hostility while Driving in Highway Traffic

The majority of TAB individuals, whether they are women or men, feel time urgent and become frequently angered by what they consider the importunate actions of other car drivers (e.g., excessive speed, tailgating, fishtailing, and close cutting in). To remedy this "traffic sickness," we have found the following regimen to be extremely effective:

1. At the initial meeting the group leader should attribute the reactions that TAB persons have to other drivers and unavoidable delays in traffic flow to the unconscious wishes of TAB persons to play the role of either God or a highway traffic officer.

2. The participant's newly formed monitor is instructed to remain alert and ready to admonish the participants if they react to any highway incident with anger or impatience.

3. Each of the participants at the second and all succeeding sessions is asked if he or she had lost patience or had become angry during his or her highway journeys between group meetings. If a participant admits that he or she had lost patience or temper at some other driver, the group leader rolls a pair of dice. The group leader notes the number the dice show and counts the participants starting with the participant who committed the highway error. When the group leader reaches the number shown on the dice, he or she stops and this innocent participant pays a fine of 5 dollars for the traffic mistake of his or her fellow participant.* Of course, the erring participant feels doubly distressed that his or her loss of patience or temper has cost a totally blameless fellow participant 5 dollars.

But this is not all that the group leader does. He also plays 5 minutes of a tape-recorded conversation in which a very severe TAB person relates how irritated and angry he or she becomes at the errors of other drivers. His/her remarks are followed by a similar conversation with a type B executive who rarely finds driving a matter for suffering temper tantrums. The contrast between the violent, almost senseless, driving reactions suffered by the TAB person and the calm, commonsense views and reactions of the type B individual is so striking that it makes the former appear not only irrational but also ridiculous.

This entire procedure, if a traffic error is reported, is repeated each session. What soon occurs is that each participant's monitor begins to warn its possessor as soon as he or she begins to drive, "Remember not to lose your 'cool,' because if you do, you'll cause another member of your group to pay a fine for your stupidity and, even worse, subject yourself and all the members of your group to listening again to that horrible tape."

Perhaps to the reader this procedure seems childish, silly, and ineffective, but the facts are that it now has been executed in over 150 groups of

*Professor Carl Thoresen of Stanford University designed this system of fines.

unsophisticated as well as ultrasophisticated individuals and the results are always the same: Within a period of 4 months (or 12 group sessions) and after an approximate 75 dollars in fines have been collected in each group, every member of all these groups no longer feels impatience or anger while driving on the highway.

One might believe, on first consideration, that participants might not admit becoming angry at a traffic incident. The group participants, however, are so eager to admit their possible lapses that they will offer traffic situations and reactions that are legitimate and reasonable. For example, more than just several times we have had to assure a participant that he or she had good reason to feel annoyed when preparing to back his or her car into a parking space, he or she observed that another driver, although aware of the participant's intent and priority, nevertheless attempted to slither his or her car, engine first, into the same parking space.

Modification of Free-Floating Hostility

In attempting to help TAB participants reduce their anger/hostility, it is important that the group leader recognize the magnitude of the task he or she is undertaking. The group leader is in fact asking them to relinquish a long-standing worldview and coping style that they previously thought was necessary for their economic or professional survival. For example, some hostile TAB persons have viewed others with suspicion and cynicism as a protection against the possible future pain of disappointment and betrayal. Others have responded with anger/hostility to even trivial situations and actions that they believe are in error. Indeed, it is a real question whether TAB persons become angry/hostile because they are not in direct control of various actions or because they perceive that these actions are being executed erroneously. In other words, would a TAB person feel anger/hostility if he or she were not in control of an event even though he or she recognized that it was being executed properly? I am not sure of the answer to this question.

Because I am essentially seeking to help TAB participants change some of their worldviews and lifelong styles of coping, intervention must focus on: (1) encouraging the individual's understanding of TAB anger/hostility; (2) promoting the individual's self-recognition of the specific causes of his or her own anger/hostility; (3) substituting new for old beliefs; (4) developing the self-monitor to prevent episodes of anger/hostility; (5) performing new habit-forming exercises; and (6) modifying angry/hostile styles of communication.

SELF-DETECTION BY TAB PARTICIPANTS OF THEIR FREE-FLOATING HOSTILITY

Initially, the specific behavioral manifestations of type A hostility (as was done for recognition of time urgency) must be comprehensively described and discussed. These manifestations (symptoms/traits and psychomotor signs) are listed in Chapter 3. I already have discussed the impatience of the type A subject when driving. But this impatience is usually accompanied by hostility. This unreasonable emotion in the majority of cases disappears when the monitor admonition–dice–tape-recording process is employed (see Chapter 6).

The presence of marital tension and competition and chronic difficulties in filial relationships are possible TAB manifestations that may not be recognized or easily admitted by many TAB persons. These are matters, however, that may emerge after a few group sessions have occurred. It has been my experience that when these familial manifestations are disclosed, they become the subjects of group discussion for an indefinite number of sessions. Similarly, the tendency of so many type A subjects to react hostilely to the trivial errors of commission and omission of their business peers and subordinates as well as their familial members is a trait that has been so well rationalized that it may take the group leader many months to induce such patients to recognize this tendency as a manifestation of their TAB disorder.

If the TAB participant is frequently unable to recognize the above traits as abnormal, he or she is even more unaware of certain psychomotor signs that he or she exhibits. For example, he or she often may be totally oblivious of possessing a laugh, voice, or both that indicate the presence of hostility. After his or her induced recognition of signs, he or she must be instructed to indulge, under the aegis of his or her self-monitor, in those exercises designed to alter these vocal indicators of hostility.

TAB subjects who exhibit upper eyelid or lateral mouth retraction tics (see Chapter 3) are almost always unaware of exhibiting these significant signs of hostility. Therefore, they must be informed both of their presence and that they cannot be obliterated by any specific exercise. They decrease in frequency of occurrence or disappear only after a general diminution of hostility takes place.

The presence of periorbital pigmentation (see Fig. 3.3), which may be a result of either a chronic sense of time urgency, free-floating hostility, or both, should not be brought to the attention of the patient. This is because I know of no exercise or drill that can do away with this corticotropin-induced variety of skin tanning.

SELF-RECOGNITION BY TAB SUBJECTS OF THE SPECIFIC INCITANTS OF THEIR FREE-FLOATING HOSTILITY

I previously have discussed the covert presence of insecurity and inadequate self-esteem that initiates, sustains, and enhances the development of TAB. Nevertheless, there often are particular or specific human actions that may intensify the ire of individual TAB persons. For example, there are many TAB subjects who become angry if, while waiting in a supermarket express lane, they observe a customer ahead of them possessing more than 10 items or someone who writes a check to pay for his or her purchases. On the other hand, there are other TAB persons who might not be angered by the preceding events but who seethe at events such as being interrupted by another when they are speaking, encountering the unrolling of toilet paper in a direction of which they do not approve, observing a frayed American flag, witnessing a person expectorating on the street, hearing a voice or laugh that is too loud, receiving a traffic violation ticket, detecting a slight grammatical error in a memorandum, and so forth. Recognition of these sorts of incidents, so often of trivial importance, is one of the first steps in the process of eliminating such arousals.

Substitution of New for Old Belief Systems

NEW BELIEF: *The intensity of a hostile reaction should be commensurate with the magnitude of the other person's error*

The group leader must encourage his or her patients to believe that anger, under certain circumstances, is a natural and legitimate emotional response to a frustration that is of major proportions or to a serious or even a moderate threat to one's security and integrity. The error in TAB is not an angry response to a truly disturbing event; it is anger that occurs more frequently at trivial incitements and that is more intense and of longer duration. One of the salient advantages of the perfected self-monitor is its capacity to gauge instantaneously the intensity and importance of a possible anger-inducing incident.

NEW BELIEF: *Most people can be trusted to act honestly and nonmalevolently*

Frequently, but by no means invariably, TAB subjects possess a hyper-critical view of both persons and things. This view of other persons as malevolent becomes understandable when one realizes that it is not difficult to downgrade other persons if one's own self-esteem is substandard.

This hostile perception of the world can be revealed sometimes by an exercise in which the group leader asks his or her participants to list all the imperfections that they can identify in the furnishings of their meeting room. After they have done this, they are asked to identify the pleasing features of the same room. From such an exercise, participants are usually struck with the ease and paradoxical pleasure with which they are able to find imperfections compared with the difficulty they encounter when they attempt to see positive qualities in this same meeting room.

NEW BELIEF: *The bestowal and receipt of praise, affection, and love always enhance, never diminish, one's self-esteem*

Much has been published about the presence of cynicism in TAB persons. Indeed, there are some who have designated it as the driving causal force of the total behavior pattern. This last concept, however, is patently incorrect because cynicism by its nature is a sequential, not an innovative, phenomenon. But cynicism, while by no means present in all TAB subjects, is more frequently observed than the ability of these same persons to praise and give affection and love to other people.

Although we have witnessed in hundreds of these subjects their reluctance to bestow praise on their business and professional peers and subordinates and most particularly to the members of their family, the causes of such reluctance are not easily discerned in all cases. Of course, it is axiomatic that if one's own self-esteem is inadequate, there must be a disinclination to praise the virtues of others. Once one becomes chronically critical of others, the expression of praise might feel quite awkward. Then, too, often, there is a downright shyness to give praise to another.

There is also the fact that since most TAB persons are married to spouses also afflicted with the TAB disorder, who are also reluctant to offer praise, the marital dispensation of this spiritually refreshing variety of communication may be minimal. Similarly, the verbalization of affection (and love) to one's spouse, children, and close friends is a difficult articulation for a large fraction of TAB individuals. Unfortunately, however, affection and love prosper on the verbalization of their existence.

The activation of this new belief does not come easily and its development must be encouraged continuously by the group leader as well as by the afflicted subject's conscientious involvement in some of the exercises specifically focused on this development (see Appendix 1). Once the TAB person begins to give praise, affection, and love, he or she in turn often begins to receive these most charming components of human intercourse. His or her sense of self-esteem certainly is never damaged by their receipt.

NEW BELIEF: *Hostility never adds to but often subverts the progress of a career*

Once enthusiasm, hard work, leadership, intellect, and creative judgment are defined and sharply differentiated from hostility or anger, it is the rare TAB person who continues to believe that his or her easily aroused anger or hostility has played a part in the advancement of his or her economic or social career.

We know of no one interventional measure that is more instrumental in diminishing the easy arousal of anger or hostility than the initial revelation that this emotion has played at best only a negative role in the course of a business or professional career. There may be rare occasions when thinking is heightened by hostility, but usually its presence impedes the recognition of one's own ideas.

NEW BELIEF: *Mysteries, doubts, and uncertainties are frequent components of normal living; they should not serve as incitants of anger*

The underlying insecurity of a TAB person encourages the arousal of irritability and aggravation when he or she encounters what John Keats described as "the uncertainties, mysteries and doubts" of life. He or she must recognize, as Keats eventually managed to do, that persons can find tranquillity even if, at times, fact and reason appear absent in various situations.

SPECIFIC APPLICATION OF SELF-MONITOR TO FREE-FLOATING HOSTILITY MANIFESTATIONS

I already have described the construction of a self-scrutinizing monitor for the instant detection and correction of feelings of inadequate self-esteem, time urgency, and impatience. This same self-monitor must also learn to recognize the symptoms and psychomotor signs of anger/hostility so that it may instantly detect and cognitively filter all external stimuli that might evoke anger/hostility.

I have found that one of the most effective measures in developing the self-monitor's efficiency in cognitively filtering out perceptions of potential anger-/hostility-inducing reactions is the employment of a particular metaphor. This consists of likening a TAB subject who surrenders to an impulsive rage reaction to a fish that, when encountering a bait carrying a barbed hook, thoughtlessly and impulsively attempts to ingest the barbed bait and hopelessly hooks itself. This metaphor of pejoratively likening a TAB

person to a fish who hooks itself (i.e., reacts with anger/hostility) on a bait
(i.e., a trivial or inconsequential gaffe of another person) was observed by
Dr. Lynda Powell in 1980 to be an extraordinarily effective tool to get easily
angered TAB persons to recognize that, far from being in emotional control
of their milieu, they respond too often to situations like a fish responds to
a bait-carrying hook.

An important means of increasing participants' understanding of their
"fish–bait–hook" reactions is to involve them in a self-monitoring exercise
in which they identify and evaluate the power of bait events or situations at
home, at work, and elsewhere. During such exercises the participants are
encouraged to evaluate the frequency, intensity, and duration of their
angry/hostile responses to various bait situations. Appendix 5 presents some
typical bait situations and the hook responses that, in the absence of a
cognitively filtering monitor, can generate anger/hostility.

The development of a self-monitor that will work rapidly and effectively in combating the arousal of anger/hostility cannot be accomplished
in a few weeks or months. Perhaps the first encouraging sign of its development is the TAB participant's recognition and self-censure after the eruption of anger/hostility in response to a trivial event. The next step in its
development occurs when the TAB participant almost responds angrily to
an event but his or her monitor "catches" him or her in time. The final stage,
of course, is reached when events evoke either no emotional response or
one of understanding, compassion, or even forgiveness, if necessary.

DAILY PERFORMANCE OF NEW
HABIT-FORMING EXERCISES

Just as exercises are recommended for the enhancement of self-esteem
and the moderation of time urgency and impatience, a set of exercises for
the alleviation of anger/hostility are also to be done on a daily basis. These
are found in Appendix 1. The same directions given for following those
exercises, designed to enhance security and self-esteem and alleviate time
urgency and impatience, also should be followed in daily pursuing those
exercises designed to alleviate easily induced, free-floating hostility. Often
the participants will bring up questions or enquire about the exercises or
more often about the significance or even the relevance of the four general
truths or principles printed at the bottom of each monthly exercise page
(see Appendix 2).

As is done for the alleviation of time urgency and impatience, group
discussions dealing with anger/hostility begin with an understanding and

memorization of the psychomotor signs indicative of free-floating hostility. Most signs should be mimicked when possible by the group counselor so that participants (and their self-monitor) easily recognize such signs when they appear in themselves.

Group leaders should encourage their participants to offer accurate but constructive and supportive feedback to other participants of the group. The group leader, however, must see to it that the suggestions of one participant to another are neither destructive nor competitive. Then, too, praising the honesty and courage of participants who are able to identify and admit their hostility is a powerful incentive to other group members to do likewise.

Because meticulously continuous self-monitoring is an unattainable ideal state, participants become aware of lapses. Such lapses, when admitted, provide the group leader with opportunities to help participants become aware of their often perfectionistic standards for change.

Even at a very early stage of treatment, the sense of self-control that results from self-monitoring rewards participants in two crucial ways. First, they acquire the ability, unlike the fish helplessly grabbing a baited hook, to choose *not* to respond. Second, by reducing their previous hostile responses in personal relationships, they lessen the interpersonal isolation that participants so often experience. These early results also enhance the self-esteem of these persons.

IDENTIFICATION OF ANGRY/HOSTILE STYLES OF COMMUNICATION

Participants, in addition to becoming skilled at instantly identifying old erroneous beliefs and provocative situations that previously triggered their anger/hostility, need to develop an increased awareness of their styles of expressing their dissent. For instance, many TAB persons express their dissent in a highly aggressive and confrontive style that they erroneously have perceived as effective. Through a more reflective examination and the honest feedback of other members of the group, such individuals begin to recognize that their prior angry/hostile mode of expressing their dissent or disagreement often precipitates an angry counterattack that prolongs and escalates angry/hostile emotions. The recognition of these prior modes of expressing dissent confronts participants with their ineffectiveness and its often staggering cost to their spouses, children, friends, colleagues, and not least to themselves.

In the group discussion of modes of expressing as well as receiving dissent or disagreement, however, participants must be warned that if anger/hostility does occur, despite the preventive efforts of their self-monitor, such anger/hostility should not be suppressed only to induce a chronic state of seething or aggravation. There are sometimes legitimate causes for anger or hostility, and when they occur, an angry or hostile reaction may be a normal response, not an indication of a medical disorder. It must be remembered that even Jesus responded angrily when he encountered the money lenders in the Temple.

8

Encouragement of Numinous Enrichment

THE DECLINE OF WESTERN RELIGIONS

There is little question that today a serious erosion has taken place in Western culture's faith or belief in the existence of either a theistic or deistic creator in his or her universe. Just what have been the major causes of this decline in the belief of a warm, guiding, protective, prayer-amenable deity are debatable. But there is little question that scientific inventions have played a significant role in this widespread decline in religious belief. Scientists insist that no agency can change the immutable play and interplay of chemical and physical reactions. Thus, there can be no miracles in our universe, and stripped of its miracles, Western religions lose their plinths of belief.

This leaves Western society a merciless, uncaring world. And the icons of contemporary materialism (e.g., computers, luxury cars, electronic gadgets of myriad varieties, jewels, ornate house furnishings, etc.) provide no spiritual support. The failure of these icons to provide even a teardrop of spiritual sustenance is the reason that the TAB person's acquisition of more and more of such ephemera fails to give him the peace and security that comes with enough. Unfortunately, too often TAB persons never learn that more never leads to enough. Such persons sooner or later must face up to the realization that to obtain peace and contentment of mind, they must enhance their spiritual qualities. This latter is not easy to accomplish if such persons have lost their belief that there is a deity that will reward them for the development of such qualities.

85

THE ENHANCEMENT OF ONE'S SPIRITUAL QUALITIES

I already have emphasized (see Chapter 5) the transcendent importance of giving and receiving affection and love not only to members of one's family but also to friends. Boiled down, the core of all Western religions is love for one's fellow person. As I also have observed earlier, it is not easy for a TAB person to learn that one true friend is more to be sought than a dozen acquaintances.

It also must be remembered that a person's regard for his or her pet and, in turn, his or her acceptance of the pet's affection is a spiritual transaction. Repeatedly, we have observed the newly found happiness our TAB participants experience after they have brought a dog or cat into their homes.

It is a truth worth pondering about that the free-floating hostility of a TAB man or woman never flares in his or her loving relationship with his or her dog or cat.

Admittedly, the absorbed reading of a fun book, the devoted listening to a splendid symphony, or the inspired inspection of a superb Renaissance painting or sculpture are not, strictly speaking, spiritual events. But they do favor the possible emergence of numinous feelings. Certainly, they are more likely to do so than the acquisition of mere things or the struggle for power.

Similarly, viewing the rising or setting of the sun, listening to the rushing of the wind through tall pine trees, and hearing the rippling of a brook or the crashing sounds of ocean waves are not per se spiritual entities, but certainly they intimate the existence of such qualities. Moreover, involvement in such phenomena of nature conceivably might encourage the spiritual growth of TAB persons.

To summarize this difficult but almost essential step toward modification of TAB, it must be admitted that it is not an easy task for the TAB person to engage in experiences whose value cannot be measured by cash register or computer. But our interventional measures can be directed toward having him or her strive to achieve transcendence beyond himself. There is no better path to those things making up a man's or woman's soul.

9

Effectiveness of Type A Counseling in Postmyocardial Infarction Patients and Normal Subjects

POSTMYOCARDIAL INFARCTION PATIENTS GIVEN TYPE A COUNSELING

Although my colleagues and I, as well as other investigators, had accumulated considerable evidence suggesting that TAB was associated with the incidence of clinical coronary heart disease in the two decades following the recognition of TAB in coronary patients in 1959, a direct, unequivocal connection between this syndrome and the pathogenesis of clinical coronary heart disease remained to be demonstrated. It was with this goal in mind that we designed a program in which a large number of patients who had suffered one or more myocardial infarctions would be randomized into two groups. The first group would be advised by cardiologists concerning well-recognized, possible preventive measures, such as cessation of smoking, ingestion of low-fat, low-cholesterol diets, adequate exercise, and other heart-related factors. The second group would be advised similarly by the same cardiologists but in addition would be given type A counseling by psychologists, psychiatrists, and several internists who had received training in type A group counseling.

This study, now well-known as the Recurrent Coronary Prevention Project (Friedman et al., 1986), was begun in 1978, supported by the

National Heart, Lung and Blood Institute, and scheduled to continue for 5 years. We were able to recruit 862 postinfarction patients in 1978 who were randomized to either a control group of 270 participants who received only group cardiac counseling or an experimental group of 592 participants who received both cardiac and TAB intervention.

The baseline sociodemographic and medical findings in both random-ized groups were essentially the same. Thus, the mean age was 53 years, approximately 90% were men, 74% had smoked cigarettes,* 39% had a history of hypertension, 39% had angina, and 25% had undergone coronary bypass surgery. Over 90% of the patients were found to exhibit TAB according to the videotaped structured interview (VSI).

All participants at entry filled out a self-report (participant question-naire) and repeated this process annually. The experimental participants (i.e., those receiving cardiac and type A counseling) also were asked to have similar questionnaires filled out by their spouses (spouse questionnaire) and by an associate at work (monitor questionnaire). These also were repeated annually.

Treatment

The 270 cardiac-counseled participants in groups of 12 were given cardiac counseling concerning a low-cholesterol, low-fat diet, adequate exercise but avoidance of severe exercise, control of possible hypertension, and announcement of any new cardiac drugs. They attended 25 group sessions of 90 minutes each over the 4.5-year period.

The 592 cardiac–type A-counseled participants were enrolled in 60 groups, each group also containing approximately 12 participants. They received the same amount of cardiac counseling as the control cardiac-counseled participants, as well as receiving TAB counseling. They attended 38 counseling sessions in their 4.5-year period of involvement.

The TAB program given to the cardiac type A participants consisted of all the procedures described previously in Chapters 5–8. A treatment failure was a participant of either group who failed to attend three counsel-ing sessions or, if a member of the second group, who failed to adopt the measures recommended by his or her TAB counselor. One hundred four (36.6%) of the cardiac-counseled and 253 (42.2%) of the cardiac–type A-counseled patients withdrew from the project during the 4.5-year period.

*All participants, however, had quit smoking for at leat 6 months prior to entry.

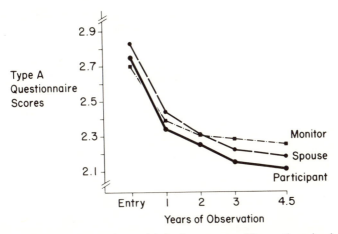

Figure 9.1. Decremental changes in type A behavior as measured by questionnaires in type A postmyocardial infarction participants given type A counseling for 4.5 years. The questionnaires were obtained yearly from a business associate (monitor), the spouse, and from the participant himself. Note that degree of behavior change observed by participants, spouses, and monitors was essentially the same. (From Friedman et al., 1986. Reprinted with permission.)

Results

We employed the Intention to Treat Principle by which we calculated the 4.5 years' results of all participants who initially entered the study if we were able to obtain their medical status at the end of the 4.5-year period. The behavioral results and the cardiac recurrence rates of these 234 cardiac-counseled patients (group 1) and 536 type A-cardiac-counseled (group 2) patients are described in the following section.

Changes in Intensity of TAB in Cardiac-Counseled and Cardiac–Type A-Counseled Participants

A marked decline in TAB occurred in the cardiac–type A-counseled patients as observed by their monitors, spouses, and themselves (see Fig. 9.1). The decline in TAB intensity was most dramatic during the first year of TAB counseling, after which it decreased further but at a far less precipitous rate.

Also, the decline in TAB as measured by the videotaped clinical examination (VCE) was quite marked 4.5 years after type A counseling had begun in the cardiac–type A-counseled participants. As Table 9.1 illustrates, 28.0 fell to 15.5 at the end of 4.5 years, a 46% fall. This fall was statistically

Table 9.1. Changes in Type A Behavior in Type A–Cardiac-Counseled and Cardiac-Counseled Patients (Controls)

	Type A–cardiac counseled patients (n = 536)			Cardiac-counseled patients (n = 235)		
	At entry[a]	4.5 years	Percent change	At entry	4.5 years	Percent change
Videotaped clinical interview	28.0 (11.9)	15.5 (8.9)[b]	−46.4	30.2 (12.4)	22.0 (9.4)[c]	−27

[a]Numerals in parentheses, standard deviation.
[b]$P < 0.0001$ vs. entry score.
[c]$P < 0.05$ vs. entry score.

significant. On the other hand, the VCE of the cardiac-counseled participants declined from the entry score of 30 to 22 when those participants were given the VCE again 4.5 years after they had entered the study. These results obtained from the cardiac–type A-counseled patient, his or her spouse, and his or her monitor, together with the VCE changes, left little doubt that a marked decline in the intensity of the TAB had been achieved in the cardiac–type A-counseled patients.

The Cardiac Recurrence Rates in the Cardiac-Counseled and Cardiac–Type A-Counseled Patients

There was no question at the end of 3 years that significant protection against a cardiac recurrence had been provided for the group of participants who had been given cardiac–type A intervention (see Fig. 9.2). Thus, at 3 years, whereas the cumulative annualized recurrence rate* was approximately 5% in the cardiac-counseled group of patients, the rate was approximately 2.5% in the cardiac–type A-counseled participants.

At the end of 4.5 years, the total cardiac recurrence rate was 12.9% in the cardiac–type A-counseled participants (see Table 9.2 and Fig. 9.2) and 21.2% in those participants given only cardiac counseling. This difference in cardiac recurrences was statistically significant.

Forty-one of the 69 recurrences in the cardiac–type A-counseled groups of patients were repeat myocardial infarctions. Thirty-three of the

*The cumulative annualized cardiac recurrence rate was determined at 3-month intervals throughout the 4.5 years. The general formula used for calculation of this cumulative annualized cardiac recurrence rate is described in Friedman et al. (1986).

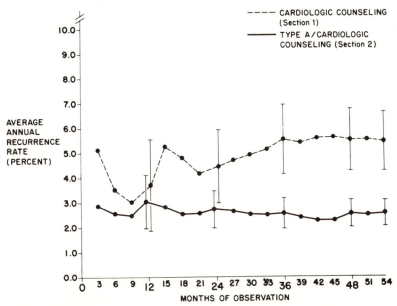

Figure 9.2.   Cumulative annualized recurrence rates in cardiac-counseled (n = 235) and type A–cardiac-counseled (n = 536) postmyocardial participants of the RCPP study. Note that 95% confidence limits of quarterly calculated recurrence rates of the two groups no longer intersect at the end of 36 months. (From Friedman et al., 1986. Reprinted with permission.)

50 recurrences in the cardiac-counseled group of participants were repeat myocardial infarctions.

At the end of the first year of the study the cardiac death rate in the two groups of patients was approximately the same. However, during the last 3 years of the 4.5-year period the cardiac death rate in the cardiac–type A-counseled patients (3.4%) was significantly less than that (6.4%) observed in the cardiac-counseled patients (see Table 9.2).

Not to our surprise, even better results were obtained in the 141 patients who had undergone coronary bypass surgery prior to their entry into the study and were given cardiac–type A counseling for 4.5 years. Their recurrence rate at the end of 4.5 years was 14.9% (see Table 9.3), less than half the recurrence rate (34.4%) observed in the 67 cardiac-counseled bypass patients. This difference, of course, was statistically significant.

On the other hand, taken as an entire group, the 208 bypass patients, compared to the remaining 563 patients who did not have coronary bypass surgery prior to entry, showed approximately the same recurrence rate at the end of 4.5 years. This failure of coronary bypass surgery alone to decrease the recurrence rate in our infarction patients agrees with the

Table 9.2. Cardiac Recurrence Rates in Type A–Cardiac-Counseled Patients and Cardiac-Counseled Patients

	Total number at risk (4.5 years)	Total recurrence (nonfatal infractions and cardiac deaths) in 4.5 years	Nonfatal infractions in 4.5 years	Cardiac deaths	
				First year	Remaining 3.5 years
Type A–cardiac-counseled patients	536	69 (12.9%)^a	41 (7.6%)^b	10 (1.7%)	18 (3.4%)^a
Cardiac-counseled patients	235	50 (21.2%)	33 (14.0%)	2 (0.8%)	15 (6.4%)

^{a}P < 0.05 vs. cardiac-counseled participants.
^{b}P < 0.02 vs. cardiac-counseled participants.

results of other previous studies in which the long-term prognosis of patients subjected to coronary bypass failed to significantly alter their long-term survival.

These therapeutic results effected in postinfarction patients by modification of their TAB and that alone, significant as they appear to be, were published in 1986 (Friedman et al., 1986). In a recent study of 268 postinfarction patients in which half were given a short course of TAB counseling, G. Burell and her associates at Uppsala University Medical School found their results were approximately the same as ours (personal communication). These will soon be published.

SUBJECTS SUFFERING FROM TAB BUT OTHERWISE HEALTHY GIVEN TYPE A INTERVENTION MEASURES FOR 8 MONTHS

In 1984, with the consent of the Research Committee of the Walter Reed Medical Center, the Surgeon General of the US Army, and the Commandant of the US Army War College, we selected 118 of the 188 lieutenant colonel students of the Army War College who had volunteered for a 9-month course of type A counseling. The 118 lieutenant colonels were those who on entry were adjudged the most type A (by questionnaire and by VSI of the original 188 who had volunteered. The 118 selected were then randomized and 62 officers were given type A counseling for 9 months and 56 officers served as controls. Each of these participants had been examined by history, physical examination, and resting and stress electrocardiography and were found to be seemingly free of cardiovascular disease.

Table 9.3. Cardiac Recurrence Rates in Type A–Cardiac-Counseled and
Cardiac-Counseled Postinfarction Bypass Patients

Type A–cardiac-counseled patients		Cardiac-counseled patients (controls)		Level of significance (P values)[a]
Number of patients	Cardiac recurrences at 4.5 years	Number of patients	Cardiac recurrences at 4.5 years	
141	21 (14.9%)	67	23 (34.4%)	0.01

[a]Comparison of recurrence rates in type A–cardiac-counseled and cardiac-counseled patients (controls).

At entry, all participants were given a special questionnaire designed to measure the intensity of their TAB pattern. Prior to their filling out this questionnaire, a briefing was conducted explaining all questions contained in the questionnaire. The same questionnaire was given again at the end of the counseling period to all participants. In addition, at the end of the 9-month course, Col. Frederick R. Drews, the War College officer in general charge of the project, devised and distributed to all participants what my colleagues and I designated the US Army War College questionnaire.

A questionnaire also was given to each of the spouses of the participants. In this questionnaire, the observed behavior as well as the physical signs of TAB were sought. All the physical signs of time urgency and free-floating hostility were explained to these spouses.

Finally, each participant was asked to choose a classmate who would observe him during the 9 months of the experiment. This observer was not to be informed of the participant's status in the study.

The five type A intervention groups were given approximately 21 sessions, beginning with weekly sessions (90 minutes) for 3 months and then every 3 weeks for the remaining period of the study. The program provided was essentially that described in the foregoing chapters.

The results were clear-cut and consistent (Gill et al., 1985) as measured by the VSI (see Fig. 9.3) where there was a 56% decline ($P < 0.0001$) in the type A-counseled participants as compared to only 14% decline in the control subjects ($P < 0.01$).

If the participant's questionnaire scores were employed as a measure of change, then here again a 23% decrease in their TAB pattern occurred in the type A-counseled patients compared to a 5% fall in the control subjects. Similarly, the spouses' questionnaires showed a 26% decline in TAB in the counseled group and only an 8% decline in TAB intensity in the control participants.

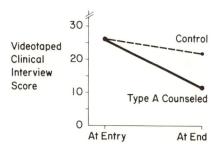

Figure 9.3.   The decremental changes at the end of 8 months in the average type A behavior of type A counseled and control officers of the US Army War College, as estimated from a comparison of the 9 months' score with the entry VSI score. (From Gill et al., 1985. Reprinted with permission.)

Also, when the student observers who had been selected by the participants were asked the following two questions at the end of the study—"Were the leadership qualities of the fellow student you observed adversely affected by their participation in the course?" and "Would you be willing to have the classmate you observed responsible for a critical component of one of your own future command organizations?"—the anonymous answer to both questions indicated that the members of the type A behavior modification groups were scored more favorably than their control counterparts.

In sum, whether judged by their improvement in just the covert and overt components of TAB or by their military qualities, the type A-counseled participants had significantly improved.

SUBJECTS GIVEN TYPE A INTERVENTION MEASURES FOR 3 YEARS

Two different groups of TAB men and women given the type A program for 3 years will be described. They are participants in our current ongoing Coronary/Cancer Prevention Project (CCPP). This study includes 3000 volunteer male and female participants (ages 45–65), who on entry appeared clinically free of both coronary heart disease and cancer (as determined by history, physical examination, and electrocardiographic and various blood studies). Half of the 3000 participants, by computer randomization, were to be given type A intervention measures for a minimum of 5 years. The remaining half received no type A counseling, but together with the type A-counseled subjects were informed every 6 or 12 months by

Table 9.4. The Changes in Type A Behavior after 3 Years of Type A Counseling

	Type A counseled subjects ($n = 233$)[a]	Type A control subjects ($n = 204$)[b]
Total VCE		
At entry	156 (56)	150 (56)
At 3 years	98 (46)	138 (51)
Percent change	−31	−7
Level of significance (*P* value)	0.0001	NS
Time urgency		
At entry	98 (38)	97 (37)
At 3 years	60 (29)	89 (34)
Percent change	−31	−5
Level of significance (*P* value)	0.0001	NS
Free-floating hostility		
At entry	58 (23)	53 (24)
At 3 years	37 (17)	49 (24)
Percent change	−24	−6
Level of significance (*P* value)	0.0007	NS
Insecurity/inadequate self-esteem		
At entry	46 (25)	44 (25)
At 3 years	31 (23)	40 (26)
Percent change	−21	−13
Level of significance (*P* value)	0.0001	NS

[a]Numerals in parentheses, standard deviation.
[b]NS, not significant.

newsletter of all recent developments occurring in prevention of coronary heart disease and cancer.

At entry, all participants were given the new VCE and scored as described in Chapter 3. They again were given the VCE after 3 years of participation in the study. The examiner both at the entry and the 3-year repeat VCE was unaware of the experimental status of any participant.

The first group consisted of 233 individuals who had been involved in the type A program for 3 years and the second group consisted of 204 control subjects who also had been in the CCPP study for the same period of time. The 233 individuals were assigned to groups (12–15 persons) and given type A intervention by the same group leader* for the 3-year period. Also, the same group leader more often than not separately counseled two or more groups.

All participants were counseled in 90-minute sessions weekly for 8 weeks, then biweekly for the remainder of the first year. They were counseled monthly during the second and third year of their participation.

*Only 11 of the 20 available leaders were involved in this part of the study.

As Table 9.4 illustrates, a statistically significant decline occurred in the total VCE (31%) and its two overt components, time urgency (31%) and free-floating hostility (24%). Also, a statistically significant decline (21%) occurred in the covert component of TAB, insecurity/inadequate self-esteem.

But as Table 9.4 also demonstrates, there was no statistically significant decline in either the total VCE or its overt and covert components in the control participants.

These marked declines in the total, overt, and covert components observed in the type A-counseled participants were amply confirmed by the general demeanor of the counseled participants. It often was difficult to believe, when the videotaped entry and 3-year examinations were compared, that it was the same individual that was being seen, so marked were the changes. Various physical signs (e.g., prolepsis, voice changes, facial grimaces, and facial hostility) in particular had diminished. Only one physical sign (periorbital pigmentation) consistently remained unchanged.

On the other hand, no clinical changes could be observed in the control participants. It was also remarkable how closely their VCE scores at the end of 3 years resembled those obtained at entry.

Concise Guide for 2-Year Course of Type A Intervention

The course during the first year will consist, at the beginning, of eight weekly sessions of 90 minutes each, followed by biweekly sessions for the rest of the year. During the second year, monthly sessions will be given. At least 12, and preferably 15, participants should comprise a group. The counseling procedures to be given at each session of the 2 years follows. Prior to opening session, all participants will be subjected to the VCE.

FIRST YEAR OF TAB COUNSELING

Session 1

1. Self-introduction of each participant: Each participant will be asked to give his or her name, business or profession, and whether he or she is married or single and the number, sex, and age of his or her children. He or she then will give his or her reason for entering the course.

2. General definition of type A and B behavior: The group leader will give a four to five sentence definition of TAB, including its subvert and overt components. He or she then will explain, using a blackboard or flip chart, that TAB in essence only comprises:

$$A = \text{Anger}$$
$$I = \text{Irritation}$$
$$A = \text{Aggravation}$$
$$I = \text{Impatience}$$

97

He or she then will differentiate this AIAI disorder from leadership qualities, good judgment, hard work or long hours, creative decisions, assertiveness, charm, and good luck.

3. Overview of counseling course (2 years):
   a. Change in belief systems: The leader will begin to substitute new belief systems for old harmful ones that should be abolished.
   b. Relaxation techniques: The leader will introduce techniques for relaxation (e.g., progressive muscular relaxation).
   c. Drills to ensure change in belief systems and harmful habits: The daily drills and philosophical concepts will be briefly described but not yet distributed by the group leader.
   d. Group discussion: Discussions for the solution of commonly encountered problems will be regularly pursued after preliminary, mostly didactic, sessions have been given.
   e. Prevention of self-destruction of personality and subsequent self-construction of personality: During the first year the group leader will concentrate on removing the harmful belief systems and habits that are working to erode the personality. Then, during the second year, he or she will concentrate mostly on constructing new behavioral habits.
   f. The acronym representing the final goal: Using the blackboard or flip chart again the group leader will write out and explain the meaning of the following acronym:

   A = Acceptance and giving of affection
   S = Serenity
   A = Acceptance of other persons' trivial errors
   S = Self-esteem enhancement

4. Ground rules: Participants will:
   a. Arrive on time and remain the entire session.
   b. Attend every session as a matter of great priority.
   c. Maintain confidentiality of group's discussions.
   d. Learn first and last names of group members as soon as possible (group leader shall expedite this process by having name cards on display during the first eight sessions).
   e. Do assigned homework.
   f. Keep and bring notebooks for every session.

5. Assignment of first three chapters of *Treating Type A Behavior and Your Heart* (Friedman & Ulmer, 1984).*

6. Closing benediction: The group leader announces that most TAB groups wish to close their session with a simple benediction. He or she then reads the following benediction:

> We are here because we realize we all need more help than we can give
>   ourselves.
> We need each other.
> So may all our efforts together be of benefit to each one.
> And may friendship or love bring enrichment to all our lives and to all
>   whose lives are in our care.
> We acknowledge this gratefully. Amen.*

After reading this, the group leader passes around a slip of paper to all participants and asks them to write "yes" or "no" as to whether they wish their group to close their sessions with either this or a similar benediction. He or she then collects the slips and asks one of the participants to read the responses as the group leader goes to the blackboard and displays the voting results. It has been my experience that, without exception, 130 groups voted to close the session with a benediction.

Session 2

1. Discussion of the assigned three chapters of *Treating Type A Behavior and Your Heart*: During this period of approximately 15 minutes, the group leader will answer any questions from the group participants about what they have read. After this discussion, he or she will assign the next three chapters to be read and then discussed at the next session.

2. Introduction of the monitor: The group leader will follow the procedure described in Chapter 5.

3. Modification of time urgency and hostility while driving in highway traffic (see Chapter 6): The group leader will come equipped with a tape that records his or her conversations first with an extreme TAB person concerning their reactions to other highway drivers; this is followed by a recorded conversation with a type B person's reactions to other highway drivers. It should not be difficult for the group leader to record such contrasting conversations. What he or she must seek to record is a TAB person whose reactions are so absurdly hostile that it almost sickens group participants to be forced to listen to it after the third or fourth time. The directions described in Chapter 6 should be followed until all participants

*The group leaders distribute this book to each participant at this first session.
*This benediction was composed for my groups by Dr. James Gill of the Jesuit Order, but any appropriate set of closing sentences may be employed.

of a group no longer become impatient or hostile in highway driving. This change is usually observed after the 12th to 15th session.

4. Determination of the absence of unconditional parental love: The group leader will follow in all its details the procedure described in Chapter 5 to find out and reveal to his or her group participants the fact that the majority of them did not receive sufficient parental love.

5. Benediction.

Session 3

1. Discussion of the three assigned chapters of *Treating Type A Behavior and Your Heart* ("The Type A Woman and the Type B Woman," "Can Type A Behavior be Modified?," "The Beginnings of a Therapeutic Revolution"). Assign next four chapters ("The Study Begins," "Results," "Who Needs Treatment," "Getting Started").

2. Repetition of the highway driving procedures (i.e., the use of dice and the listening to the taped conversations of the TAB and TBB persons if one or more participants have lost their tempers while driving).

3. Inquiry about use of monitor: Group leader asks participants to describe specific events of impatience or hostility that were detected and corrected by their monitor.

4. The group leader will give a lecture on the psychopathological characteristics and the neurological and hormonal dysfunctions of TAB: The group leader will occupy the rest of the session discussing the psychopathological characteristics, the neurological dysfunctions, and the hormonal dysfunctions of TAB. In addition, he or she will discuss the abnormal metabolism of cholesterol and triglyceride that often occurs in the presence of TAB. These subjects are described in Chapter 1. This lecture has, as its chief goal, the explanation of how TAB can lead to the premature onset of coronary heart disease, hypertension, or migraine. In this lecture the epidemiological evidence connecting TAB to the premature onset of coronary heart disease or hypertension should be discussed (for such epidemiological data, consult Friedman & Rosenman, 1959; Friedman et al., 1958, 1986; Haynes et al., 1980).

5. Benediction.

Session 4

1. Discussion of assigned chapters and assignment of next three chapters ("Alleviating Your Sense of Time Urgency," "Alleviating Your Free-Floating Hostility," "Alleviating Your Self-Destruct Tendency").

2. Repetition of the highway driving procedure.

3. Enquiry about the growing employment of their monitor.

4. Distribution and demonstration by group leader of the manifestations of TAB: The group leader will distribute, explain, and illustrate a list of all the TAB manifestations as described in Chapter 6. The participants are expected to memorize all the traits and physical signs of TAB so that within 5 minutes of encountering most persons, he or she will be capable of determining their behavioral status.

5. Benediction.

Session 5

1. Discussion of assigned chapters and assignment of next and final three chapters ("How to Avoid a Heart Attack," "Can You Modify Your Type A Behavior?," "Once More Before We Leave").

2. Repetition of the highway driving procedure.

3. Introduction of a 10-minute period of progressive muscular relaxation or its equivalent with the aim of encouraging group participants to employ the same procedure at least once daily.

4. Inquiry of individual participants to describe specific incidents in which they employed their monitor. Ask each participant if their monitors are being used five to six times daily. Encourage them to do so. The group leader gives specific examples in which his or her own monitor came into play.

5. Benediction.

Session 6

1. Discussion of the last three chapters of the book.

2. Repetition of the highway driving procedure.

3. Presentation and discussion of substitution of new for old belief systems for enhancement of self-esteem (see Chapter 5).

4. Inquiry of individual participants to relate specific incidents at which his or her monitor intervened.

5. Benediction.

Session 7

1. Presentation and discussion of substitution of new for old belief systems to modify sense of time urgency (see Chapter 6).

2. Repetition of highway driving procedure.

3. Progressive muscular relaxation.

4. Inquiry of individual participants to relate specific incidents at which their monitor intervened.

5. Benediction.

Session 8

1. Presentation and discussion of substitution of new for old belief systems to modify free-floating hostility (see Chapter 7).

2. Repetition of the highway driving procedure.

3. Showing of all participant VCE's to group: The TAB manifestations of each participant will be pointed out by the group leader.

4. Benediction.

NOTE: Sessions henceforth will be given biweekly.

Session 9

1. Introduction of drills to (1) enhance self-esteem (see Chapter 5 and Appendices 1–4), (2) modify sense of time urgency (see Chapter 6 and Appendices 1–4), and (3) modify free-floating hostility (see Chapter 7 and Appendices 1–4). The different drills listed in Appendix 1 for enhancement of self-esteem or for modification of sense of time urgency or free-floating hostility will be combined in one list containing the days of the week, and at the bottom of each monthly calendar four of the general truths or principles (obtained from Appendix 4) will be printed. One of the combined drills will be printed for each day of the week. The completed monthly calendar should look like the one illustrated in Appendix 2. Each month a new weekly list of exercises will be followed (for further explanation, see Chapter 5). A 1-year's monthly calendar, each containing 1 week's list of drills, will be distributed to the group participants and full instructions, as described in Chapter 5, will be given by the group leader.

2. Repetition of highway driving procedure.

3. Inquiry of individual participants to relate specific incidents at which his or her monitor intervened.

4. Discussion of absolute need for prioritization of daily activities with this formula to be written on blackboard and forever remembered:

$$\text{Time urgency is determined by: } \frac{\text{Number of events accepted}}{\text{Number of events avoided}}$$
$$\text{(prioritization)}$$

Participants should be told that time urgency can only be diminished by reducing this ratio.

5. Benediction.

Session 10

1. Inspection of drill books of individual participants: Each drill performed should be checked.

NOTE: There is a tendency, particularly as time elapses, for participants to no longer check that they have done an exercise. The group leader should insist that such checks should continue because it is the only way for the leader to be certain that the exercises are being done.

2. Progressive muscular relaxation.

3. Repetition of highway driving procedure.

4. Explanation of determinants of self-esteem:

$$\text{Self-esteem in part depends upon the ratio: } \frac{\text{Achievements}}{\text{Expectations}}$$

NOTE: If expectations remain too high, no matter how many achievements are accomplished, the ratio may remain low.

5. Benediction.

Session 11

1. Examination of drill books to be certain that drills are being followed.

2. Repetition of the highway driving procedure.

3. Reading of the following William James (1890, pp. 120–127) quotation:

In Professor Bain's chapter on "The Moral Habits" there are some admirable practical remarks laid down. Two great maxims emerge from the treatment. The first is that in the acquisition of a new habit, or the leaving off of an old one, we must take care to launch ourselves with as strong and decided an initiative as possible. Accumulate all the possible circumstances which shall reinforce the right motives; put yourself assiduously in conditions that encourage the new way, make engagements incompatible with the old; take a public pledge, if the case allow; in short, envelope your resolution with every aid you know. This will give your new beginning such momentum that the temptation to break down will not occur as soon as it otherwise might; and every day during which a breakdown is postponed adds to the chances of it not occurring at all.

The second maxim is, never suffer an exception to occur till the new habit is securely rooted in your life. Each lapse is like the letting fall of a ball of string which one is carefully winding up; a single slip undoes more than a great many turns will wind up again. Continuity of training is the great mean making the nervous system act infallibly right. As Professor Bain says, "The peculiarity of the moral habits, contradistinguishing them from the intellectual acquisitions, is the presence of the two hostile powers, one to be gradually raised in the ascendant over the other. It is necessary above all things, in such a situation, never to lose a battle. Every gain on the wrong side undoes the effect of many conquests on the right. The essential precaution, therefore, is to so regulate the two opposing powers that the one may have a series of uninterrupted successes, until repetition has fortified it to such a degree as to enable it to cope with the opposition, under any circumstances. This is the theoretically best career of mental progress."

4. Benediction.

Session 12

1. Exposure of the group to a type B successful individual: The group leader should invite a type B person to visit his or her group. To avoid criticisms of the group, this individual should hold a high position that was earned and is usually considered to be one associated with high stress and competition. During the type B person's visit, his or her failure to exhibit any of the traits or the physical signs of TAB should be brought to the attention of the group at the next session. Also, his or her general philosophy should be elicited and his or her high sense of self-esteem should be brought out by the group counselor, again to be commented upon in a subsequent session. I have also obtained taped interviews of type B successful men and played them to our groups. The purpose of this entire procedure is to contradict the usual TAB concept that no successful man or woman can ever be type B.
2. Benediction.

Session 13

1. Discussion of the absence of physical signs and traits of TAB in the visitor from Session 12.
2. NOTE: It should no longer be necessary to repeat the highway driving procedure because usually all participants at this juncture no longer become impatient or hostile while driving on the highway.
3. Progressive muscular relaxation.

4. Invitation to participants to present any of their own problems or views to other members of group.

5. Inspection of drill books of various participants and discussion of the four general truths or principles printed in drill book.

6. Benediction.

Session 14

1. Inquiry of individual participants to relate specific incidents in which their monitor intervened.

2. Listening to a hostile type A voice: The group leader will play the tape of a hostile type A person speaking for a few minutes followed by a type B person speaking for a few minutes. The group leader will prepare this tape by recording both a type A person with a hostile voice and type B person possessing a very pleasant voice. This tape introduces group leader's discussion about the importance of a pleasing voice.

3. Benediction.

Session 15

1. Inspection of drill books of various participants: Again, group leader emphasizes that the really effective factors in modifying TAB are the growth of participant's monitor and the exercises/drills.

2. Discussion of being verbose and the art of listening:
   a. Emphasize the tendency of TAB to indulge in being verbose.
   b. Point out that the trait of a good conversationalist is the ability to listen interestedly.
   c. To avoid excessive talking, introduce the three-question test: (1) Do I really have something important or interesting to say? (2) Is this the time to say it? (3) Does anyone wish to hear it? If the answer is "No" to any of these three questions, keep quiet.

3. Benediction.

Session 16

1. Review of all new belief systems (see Chapters 5–8).
2. Progressive muscular relaxation.
3. Discussion of group participants' problems.
4. Benediction.

Session 17

    1. Causes of success and failure: Have each participant go to the blackboard or flip chart and list (1) the causes of his or her major success, and (2) the causes of his or her greatest failure. Group leader to point out that the causes for individual successes were never due to AIAI (anger–irritability–aggravation–impatience), but that in most cases of failure, AIAI played a part.
    2. Benediction.

Session 18

    1. Continuation of investigation of causes of successes and failures begun in Session 17.
    2. Inspection of drill books of various participants.
    3. Benediction.

Session 19

    1. Discussion by the group of the four general truths or principles printed in their drill book.
    2. Inquiry of individual participants to relate specific incidents in which their monitor intervened.
    3. Group discussion of "individual" problems.
    4. Benediction.

Session 20

    1. Diagram of four circles representing thoughts, imagination, emotions, and will.
        a. Discuss imagination and will as keys to ameliorate type A behavior.
        b. Group leader explains that there are two types of energy: (1) the energy to run faster and faster in the same ditch (this is inclination of type A expenditure of energy), and (2) the energy to climb out of a ditch and make new furrows (this energy depends on the imagination and the will phases of the personality).
    2. Progressive muscular relaxation.
    3. Benediction.

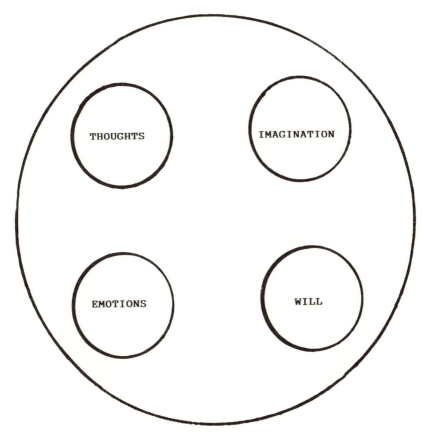

Session 21

    1. Inspection of drill books of individual participants.
    2. Reemphasis of necessity of will to begin and continue new habits.
    3. Introduction of the new fish–bait–hook metaphor (follow instructions as described in Chapter 7).
    4. Benediction.

Session 22

    1. Group discussion of new beliefs listed in Chapter 7.
    2. Progressive muscular relaxation.
    3. Suggestions to reduce time urgency:
        a. Prioritization to eliminate trash events.
        b. Purposeful overestimation of how long events will take.

c. Insertion of idle time periods in schedule.

d. Employment of will to say "no" to extraneous demands.

e. Succinct speech with total elimination of pleonasm.

4. Inspection of drill books of individual participants.

5. Request for perceived type A deficiencies: Ask participants to list their own perceived type A deficiencies that they wish to change and to bring the list in for next session's discussion period.

6. Benediction.

Session 23

1. Group discussion of each participant's list of deficiencies. To continue for Session 24 also.

2. Inquiry of individual participants to relate specific incidents in which the monitor intervened.

3. Benediction.

Session 24

1. Continuation of discussion begun in Session 23 concerning type A deficiencies.

2. Progressive muscular relaxation.

3. Request for participants to bring to the next session a list of ten things they like about themselves.

4. Benediction.

Session 25

1. Group discussion of each participant's fine qualities. Counselor should point out during this discussion that frequent recall of their fine qualities will serve to enhance self-esteem.

2. Inspection of drill books of individual participants.

3. Benediction.

Session 26

1. Group discussion of fine qualities of each participant.

2. Progressive muscular relaxation.

3. Benediction.

Session 27

1. Discussion of Karl Popper's "Three Worlds":*
   a. The physical world
   b. The world of conscious acts
   c. The world of the human mind

The group leader will facilitate a group discussion of the activities that comprise the world of the human mind. These activities include (1) memories, (2) books, (3) art and music, and (4) affection and love. It is these activities, mostly executed by the right brain, for which most TAB persons do not have time.

2. Review of each participant's initial goals for changes in habits, beliefs, and so on. (What changes have been made? What changes remain to be accomplished?)

3. Benediction.

SECOND YEAR OF TAB COUNSELING

Specific goals for second year are:

1. Review and continuation of first year drills as well as introduction of second year drills: The group leader is expected to choose specific drills or construct new drills according to the leader's observations of the needs of his or her participants.

2. Increased emphasis on and expansion of self-monitor (self-monitor to be stressed not just as a pleasant tool but one that may be vital to the participant's future physical as well as vocational integrity). These are some activities that require surveillance by self-monitor:

   a. Increased listening to and remembrance of speech of family, friends, and business associates.
   b. Speed of self-speech not to exceed 125 words/minute; also satisfactory decibel intensity of self-speech.
   c. Self-scrutiny and detection of internal tension as suggested by: (1) tension of jaw or frontal or posterior neck muscles; (2) teeth grinding; (3) knee jiggling; (4) increased expiratory sighs; and (5) failure to move diaphragm easily and smoothly when breathing.
   d. Observation of and interest in three Ps (persons, pets, and plants);

*Karl Popper, *The Poverty of Historicism,* Rutledge & Kegan Paul, London, 1961.

    e. Substitution of compassion, pity, and forgiveness for anger and hostility at trivial or unavoidable errors of other persons.

    f. Pleonastic and proleptic self-activities.

    g. Impatience.

    h. Verbalization of affection and compliments to family members, friends, associates, superiors, and subordinates.

    i. Differentiation of trash from important events or activities.

    j. No advice to family members, friends, or associates concerning their possible TAB.

3. Relaxation exercises.

4. Application of recently, as well as already learned, anti-AIAI coping measures to contemporary problems:

    a. All individual problems that are discussed should have relevance to total group.

    b. As individual problems are discussed, group leader should continuously scan all group members to observe their reactions to the airing of individuals' problems. If one or more members show boredom or restlessness, the discussion of an individual's problem should be terminated as soon as possible.

    c. Every effort should be made to involve each participant at least once per session.

5. Continued encouragement of group cohesion.

6. Enhancement of peace of mind through:

    a. Encouragement of increased interest in arts, literature, music, etc.

    b. Increased awareness of past and present accomplishments.

    c. Realistic reassessment of vocational goals to be sure that their attainment lies within the paradigm of the probable.

7. Be sure to prepare for each session. At its beginning, never fail to announce what will be discussed during that session and, at the end, always summarize briefly what transpired during the session. Urge participants to note what had transpired and continue to review their activities. (Note: One of the most frequent criticisms voiced by participants about their group leader is that he or she does not appear to have prepared for sessions or that the sessions seemed poorly organized or directed.)

8. The second VCE score is to be divided into three score categories of 400–150, 149–100, and 99–0, which represent very severe TAB, severe TAB, and moderate to no TAB, respectively. Each of these three score categories describe quantitatively the intensity of any TAB manifestation or reaction. The intensity of 11 TAB-related or influenced activities has been graded into these three score categories. One of the 11 TAB-influ-

enced activities will be discussed for 10–30 minutes at each of the first 11 counseling sessions.

The purpose of this three-score category procedure is to provide participants with (1) an understanding of their VCE score in terms of the intensity of their TAB manifestations and reactions and (2) TAB manifestations of their own that still need to be diminished in their intensity.

Session 1

1. Approaches to parenting

VCE SCORE = 400–150
  a. Irritable insistence on children's perfectionism.
  b. Frequent stream of criticisms and avoidance of compliments for fear that the latter may subvert the effectiveness of a future criticism; that is, a disbelief that one can effectively criticize at one time and compliment at another time.
  c. No enthusiastic interest and curiosity about the contents of school or college courses taken by children.
  d. A positive reluctance to embrace, hug, or kiss his or her children even though there is no reluctance to pet or even "baby talk" to his or her pet in front of his or her children.
  e. A chronic tendency to give lectures (often repetitious) to the children.
  f. No scheduled time in which a participant can enjoy events with his or her children.
  g. Rarely do the children see or hear the participant discuss a play, a work of art, a symphony, or great historical events.

VCE SCORE = 149–100
  a. No significant improvement in errors a, c, and g listed above.
  b. Less criticism but still great difficulty in giving spontaneously felt compliments to children.
  c. Still considerable difficulty in hugging or kissing children but able to pat on shoulder or arms.
  d. Many fewer lectures to children.
  e. Occasional but no regularly scheduled time to enjoy events with children.
  f. Beginning interest in school subjects studied by children.

VCE SCORE = 99–0
   a. Absolute perfection no longer demanded of children.
   b. No criticism or unasked for advice given to children over 14 years
      of age. However, general principles of good conduct insisted
      upon with well-defined penalties for infractions.
   c. Total elimination of all lectures by acts of self-exemplification; for
      example, courtesy and amiability exemplified by participant's
      attitude to spouse.
   d. Scheduled time for children (if they wish it).
   e. Ability to give verbal and physical signs of affection. For example,
      the use of the word "love" can be employed without embarrassing
      participant or his children.

   2. Distribution of exercise/drills for second year. (See Chapter 5 and
Appendix 1 for instructions concerning second year exercises.)
   a. Participants are informed that the seven weekly exercises contain
      new exercises as well as first-year exercises.
   b. Emphasize again the importance of employing will to continue
      to regularly do exercises.

   3. Distribution and discussion of the list of activities to enhance the
surveillance of self-monitor.
   4. Benediction.

Session 2

1. Social interactions

VCE Score = 400–150
   a. Style is one of unconscious hostility and dominance in voice,
      facial expression, and gestures.
   b. Listening to others is almost a painful experience. Finds it
      difficult not to interrupt speech of others.
   c. Voice often too loud, too commanding.
   d. Often approaches too near the face of others when speaking to
      them, even so close that his or her spittle showers listener or his
      or her bad breath can be smelled (at least 25% of men and women
      have halitosis).

VCE Score = 149–100
   a. Beginning to understand the depth of her/his competitive,
      domineering spirit.

    b. Recognizes that he or she has rationalized the domineering, competitive attitudes by believing that he or she is correct in his or her beliefs and actions.

    c. Begins to realize that she/he has lost the very important skill of joyful, interested listening. In other words, she/he is an impaired listener.

    d. Begins to ask others for feedback concerning his or her general behavior. Accepts even critical comments as friendly aid.

VCE Score = 99–0

    a. Voice is now pleasant and has lost its loudness, hostility, stridency, and three-alarm fire sense of time urgency.

    b. No longer requires monitor to help in listening to others because she/he now finds interest, pleasure, and a sense of acquiring knowledge in the act of listening to other persons.

    c. Laugh is modulated and no longer is too explosive.

    d. Has learned the striking effect of giving small, unexpected gifts or remembering some of the important events occurring in the lives of peers, subordinates, friends, and acquaintances.

    e. Recognizes and accepts the generally true fact that the strongest praise of his or her personality will not be heard directly by him or her but discussed among his or her subordinates, peers, superiors, acquaintances, and friends.

2. Enhancement of right-brain activities:

    a. Roger Sperry won the Nobel prize in 1981 for discovering the predominance of the left hemisphere over the "silent" right cerebral hemisphere. The activities of the left brain are predominantly concerned with numbers and words and the right brain with such activities as music, poetry, the arts, appreciation of colors, and abstruse thinking. Most TAB persons are inclined to indulge almost entirely in left-brain activities. This appears to result in the disuse and functional atrophy of those functions commonly attributed to the right brain.

    b. The group leader will inform his or her participants of the above paragraph. The leader then will designate such functional atrophy of the right brain Darwinism. This designation is justified by the leader reading the following excerpt from Darwin's (1903) letter*

*More Letters of Charles Darwin, edited by Francis Darwin, John Murray, London, 1903.

Up to the age of thirty or beyond it, poetry of many kinds gave me a great pleasure, and even as a schoolboy I took intense delight in Shakespeare, especially in the historical plays. I have also said that pictures formerly gave me considerable and music very great delight. But now for many years I cannot endure to read a line of poetry. I have tried lately to read Shakespeare, and found it so intolerably dull that it nauseated me. I have also almost lost my tast for pictures or music ... my mind seems to have become a kind of machine for grinding general laws out of large collections of facts; but why this should have caused the atrophy of that part of the brain alone, on which higher tastes depend, I cannot conceive .... If I had to live my life again, I would have made a rule to read some poetry and listen to some music at least once every week; for perhaps the part of my brain now atrophied would thus have been kept alive to use. The loss of these tastes is a loss of happiness, and may possibly be injurious to the intellect, and more probably to the moral character, by enfeebling the emotional part of our nature. (p. 36)

The group leader, after reading this to the group, points out that Darwin was correct in believing that a center in his brain had "atrophied" in that a part of the brain not used is like a leg muscle in a plaster cast: It tends to wither from disuse. The group leader further illustrates what happens to the right brain when the left brain, with its focus on facts, numbers, and so on, predominates by reading the following excerpt from Mark Twain's (1982) autobiography in which he describes his training to be a pilot on a Mississippi steamboat:*

Now when I had mastered the language of this water and had come to know every trifling feature that bordered the great river as familiarly as I knew the letters of the alphabet, I had made a valuable acquisition. But I had lost something, too. I had lost something that could never be restored to me while I lived. All the grace, the beauty, the poetry had gone out of the majestic river!

But as I have said, a day came when I began to cease from noting the glories and the charms which the moon and the sun and the twilight wrought upon the river's face; another day came when I ceased altogether to note them.

No, the romance and the beauty were all gone from the river. All the value any feature of it had for me now was the amount of usefulness it could furnish toward compassing the safe piloting of a steamboat. Since those days, I have pitied doctors from my heart. What does the lovely flush in a beauty's cheek mean to a doctor but a "break" that ripples above some deadly disease? Are not all her visible charms sown thick with what are to him signs and symbols of hidden decay? Does he ever see her beauty at all, or doesn't he simply view her professionally, and comment upon her un-

*Mark Twain, *Life on the Mississippi*, The Library of America, New York, 1982.

wholesome condition all to himself? And doesn't he sometimes wonder whether he has gained most or lost most by learning his trade? (p. 217)

c. After the Twain excerpt is read and the loss of right-brain activity is discussed by the group leader and the participants, the group leader reads an excerpt of C. G. Jung (1918) from his book, *Memories, Dreams, Reflections*:

> As a matter of fact, day after day we live far beyond the bounds of our consciousness; without our knowledge, the life of the unconscious is also going on within us.
> The more the *critical reason dominates, the more impoverished life becomes*; but the more of the unconscious and the more of the myth we are capable of making conscious, the more of life we integrate. Overvalued reason has this in common with political absolutism, under its dominion the individual is pauperized.
> The unconscious helps by communicating things to use or making figurative allusions. (p. 62)

d. Initiation of reading of (1) essays of Montaigne,* and (2) essays of Emerson (1981)† with the object of illustrating to them the severe functional atrophy of their own right brain. Thus, they should be forewarned of the difficulty that they will encounter in reading these essays because of their own "Darwinism." One group participant will read a Montaigne essay and another participant will read an Emerson essay. They are to report at their next session the thesis of the essay in 3–5 minutes. After this report, the essay will be discussed for 5–10 minutes by other group participants.

3. Benediction.

Session 3

1. Relation to time

VCE Score = 400–150
   a. Feels "squeezed," rushed, feeling there is never enough time.
   b. Finds it very difficult to say "no" to new involvements (lacks courage to respond negatively because he or she "hears" that the suppliant will think less of him or her).

---

*Montaigne, M., *Essays*, Penguin Books, New York, NY, 1958.
†Emerson, R. W., *The Portable Emerson*, Penguin Books, New York, NY, 1981.

    c. Employs polyphasic actions in preference to single acts.
    d. Fearful of delegation.
    e. Uses the hope of "some day" as a Band-Aid.

VCE Score = 149–100
    a. Attempts to say "no" more frequently.
    b. Finds unexpected pleasure when gaps in his or her life schedule accidentally take place.
    c. Begins to wonder whether it is possible to ever make a friend of time.

VCE Score = 99–0
    a. Begins to adopt a weekly schedule in which essential priorities are first scheduled regardless of their tediousness; after priorities are scheduled, the ephemeral, trivial, and routine events are scheduled. This avoids sense of time urgency because the important activities will be done.
    b. Saying "no" is now a fixed habit.
    c. Patience becomes a pleasurable relief from impatience.
    d. Weekly scheduling of priorities allows time to be free from its involvement in trash or ephemeral events. It is this freedom of time from his or her prior enslavement to it in executing the trivial events and activities that now allows time to become a friend.
  2. Progressive muscular relaxation.
  3. Report by Montaigne and Emerson essay readers followed by general discussion of essays by group.
  4. Inspection of drill book of various participants.
  5. Benediction.

Session 4

  1. Role of monitor

VCE Score = 400–150
    a. No real conviction of the effectiveness of the monitor.
    b. Continuous neglect of employment of monitor.

VCE Score = 149–100
    a. Occasional employment of monitor.
    b. Remembrance of what monitor could have prevented had it been used.

VCE Score = 99–0

    a. Routine employment of monitor five to six times or more per day in matters of forestalling outbreak of hostility and time urgency, indulging in listening better, expressing affection, and so forth.

    b. Belief and trust in effectiveness of using monitor.

2. Report by Montaigne and Emerson essay readers followed by general discussion of essays by group.

3. Inquiry of individual participants to relate specific incidents in which his or her monitor intervened.

4. Benediction.

Session 5

1. Insecurity/inadequate self-esteem

VCE Score = 400–150

    a. Sense of security and adequate self-esteem essentially dependent on external world and based on continuous evaluation by others.

    b. Positive evaluation by peers or subordinates is not appreciated and even positive evaluation by superiors is only provisionally supportive.

    c. Negative evaluation, however, regardless of its source, is always upsetting, requiring a super effort to restore one's balance.

    d. Security and adequate self-esteem is feeling that one is in the very topmost winner's circle, but even at this apex there is a feeling that slippage may take place at any time.

    e. Employment of recall of past victories or achievements. The future fear of failure blots out the memory of past achievements.

VCE Score = 149–100

    a. Intellectually understands that sense of security/adequate self-esteem may be enhanced by recall of past achievements but emotionally still cannot act upon it.

    b. Agrees that the "things worth being" should provide more self-esteem than the "things worth having," but still prefers to use his or her energy in acquiring those things that he or she believes worth having.

    c. Finds it difficult to resort to enumeration when he or she thinks of the "things worth being." She/he has grown accustomed to evaluating everything in terms of numbers.

VCE Score = 99–0
   a. Begins to realize that his or her sense of adequate self-esteem cannot be enhanced by acquisition but only by absolute integrity, the affection that he or she gives and receives and the frequent active recall of past achievements and episodes of happiness and joy.
   b. Understands that even a sense of security is only dependent acquisition to the point of self-sustenance. Once past this point, the search for security by the acquisition of more things is only fool's play.

2. Report by Montaigne and Emerson essay readers followed by general discussion of essays by group.

3. Review of TBB (see Chapter 1–3): Group counselor should describe all the manifestations of type B, emphasizing the adequacy of their self-esteem.

4. Benediction.

Session 6

1. Personal views of the change process

VCE Score = 400–150
   a. I'm really OK, but to keep my spouse happy I'll give this course a try.
   b. I'm not sure I'll ever feel comfortable or relaxed on the highway but it's fun watching and listening to the group leader attempt to get us to enjoy commuting.
   c. I don't believe I need much change.

VCE Score = 149–100
   a. Doing these drills may be of some value and doing them doesn't do me any harm. I can see what they are trying to do.
   b. People are noticing changes in me. I'm surprised at some of their comments.
   c. Maybe I have been too hard on the family.

VCE Score = 99–0
   a. It is good to know that I needed changes and have made those changes.
   b. Life has become a sort of recovery and discovery process.
   c. I now really do have a good feeling about my self-esteem.

2. Report by Montaigne and Emerson essay readers followed by general discussion of essays by group.

3. Group discussion of any current problems encountered by individual participants. Female participants are more reticent to discuss their personal problems and the group leader must encourage them more than male participants in this regard.

4. Inspection of drill books of various participants.

5. Benediction.

Session 7

1. Responses to possible hooks and unexpected events

VCE Score = 400–150
    a. Life is a continuous series of rapid responses to situations that too often are perceived as crises or urgent matters that require immediate attention.
    b. Trivial actions of others present situations that serve as "hooks" to participants, leading to irritation or outright hostility.

VCE Score = 149–100
    a. Monitor beginning to apply the question, "Is this sort of urgent living really worthwhile?"
    b. Monitor beginning to modulate "all-out" responses or even no response to increasing number of situations.

VCE Score = 99–0
    a. Monitor immediately recognizes certain situations that previously would serve as a hook and are instantaneously neutralized by common sense.
    b. Monitor appraises all situations and detects, eliminates, or postpones various events using perspective as scale for action or no action.

2. Report by Montaigne and Emerson essay readers followed by general discussion by group.

3. Encouragement of right-brain activities by group leader: Participants are asked to involve themselves in one or more right-brain activities during the next month, such as (1) reading a book of high quality, (2) visiting a museum or gallery, or (3) attending a symphony, ballet, or drama.

4. Review of family relationships.

5. Review of changes in their old belief systems: The group leader asks participants what have been their changes in their belief systems.
6. Benediction.

Session 8

1. TAB's supposed role in vocational success

VCE Score = 400–150
   a. Absolute reluctance to separate TAB from such success entities as hard work, long hours, sustained drive, enthusiasm, creative ideas, foresight, and wisdom.
   b. Insists that most of his or her seemingly successful acquaintances exhibit TAB.
   c. Strange failure to recognize those acquaintances who are successful but exhibit TBB.
   d. Shies away from attributing past mistakes to impatience and/or easily aroused hostility.

VCE Score = 149–100
   a. Still insists that all his or her acquaintances are TAB and that TBB persons are dull and mediocre.
   b. Beginning to admit an occasional mistake due to impatience or hostility.
   c. Still peculiarly reluctant to admit knowing any TBB acquaintances, although she/he admits that they may exist.
   d. Still finding it difficult to refuse invitations to expend his or her time. Wishes to be considered nice, at all cost.

VCE Score = 99–0
   a. Increasing recognition that whatever success he or she has attained, it has not been due to AIAI but in spite of these afflictions.
   b. Beginning to make a "friend of time" by resolutely refusing to give priority to any event or self-participation unless it is of lasting value to his or her vocational or avocational activities.
   c. Growing awareness of the inverse ratio between his or her self-centeredness and his or her self-esteem.
   d. Reluctant but beginning recognition and admiration of TBB persons.

    e. Recognizes albeit slowly that TAB is always a self-destructive disease.

    f. Increasing use of monitor.

    g. Increasing recognition and compassion for the impatience and easily aroused hostility he or she sees in his or her TAB acquaintances.

2. Usual report by Montaigne and Emerson essay readers followed by general discussion by group.

3. Enquiry of participants' right-brain activities as prescribed in previous session.

4. Benediction.

Session 9

1. Approaches to the numinous

VCE Score = 400–150

    a. Distaste of organized religions or if religious is quite doctrinaire.

    b. Disinclination to "waste time" thinking about religious matters.

    c. Belief that the liturgy as well as the litany of organized religions are boring and possibly nonsensical.

    d. When you're dead, that's it!

    e. A belief that scientists are right in believing that there is no God and that chance vis-à-vis evolution has been responsible for all living entities.

    f. Most people, at best, are concerned only with themselves.

VCE Score = 149–100

    a. Participant still entertains the same beliefs regarding items a, c, and e above.

    b. Finds time at least to begin to think about whether there are forces at play not only for evil but also for good.

    c. Participant is still certain that when you die, that is the end, but finds that he or she wistfully envies those who believe there is an afterlife.

    d. Participant begins to look about him- or herself and realizes that the majority of persons are essentially good-hearted and decent.

    e. Participant begins to recognize the impossibility of understanding any facet of a multidimensional universe with his or her barely three-dimensional mind.

VCE Score = 99–0

    a. Participant becomes increasingly certain that there must be some force or forces responsible for the creation of the universe and the evolutionary creation of the finely devised myriad of chemical and physical processes that make up the structures of all living things including ourselves; that chance alone or chaos could not be this force or forces.

    b. The participant becomes consciously aware and thankful for what the now-dead have left us: not only our literature, our paintings, our great works of music, our modes of transportation and communication, but also our mundane streets and highways and many of our houses were built by persons now dead. The legacy to be left by the participant will be his or her work, children, and those inspiring contributions that can be given to his or her friends. Even the planting of a tree may be a greater legacy than the acquisition of a million dollars in stocks and bonds.

    c. The participant is convinced that whatever kind of soul he or she possesses, it can only be preserved by enhancing the lot of others.

    d. The participant finally realizes that no number exists that is capable of delighting his or her soul. Certainly the strength of love cannot be expressed by any numeral.

    e. The participant fully understands and believes the truth of the following statement by Eliot (1982): "For the growing good of the world is partly dependent on *unhistoric* acts; and that things are not so ill with you and me as they might have been, is half owing to the number who lived faithfully a hidden life and rest in unvisited tombs."

2. Usual report by Montaigne and Emerson essay readers followed by general discussion by group.

3. Request by group counselor for a general discussion of what plans each participant will make after the course ends to avoid relapses in behavior. Counselor will emphasize the role of the monitor in preventing possible relapses.

4. Benediction.

Session 10

1. Relation to friendship

VCE Score = 400–150

    a. No time or real interest in persons as "friends."

   b. Acquaintances are substitutes for friends. Acquaintances are cultivated for self-centered interests such as: (1) access to privilege, (2) advancement of career, (3) geographic proximity, and (4) heedless networking. "Friends" are always event-specific.
   c. It's not necessary to remember the names or sexes of children of acquaintances.

VCE Score = 149–100
   a. Beginning to make some discrimination between "friends" and acquaintances.
   b. A wistful but not too definite desire to make the effort to find several "friends."
   c. Wonders which of his or her acquaintances will find the time or the desire to attend his or her funeral.

VCE Score = 99–0
   a. "By God, I have made a new friend! I know his or her children, their names, his or her spouse's name. I'm interested in his or her career and he or she is in mine."
   b. I show my affection in part by asking for some of my friend's time.
   c. He or she knows that he or she is on my small list of friends because I have told him or her this.
   d. "I now recognize that the giving and receiving of affection is one of the major sources of my happiness in life."
   e. "I am beginning to try to evaluate what fraction of my fortune, as it is, I would give to save, if necessary, my best friend's life."

   2. Usual report by Montaigne and Emerson essay readers followed by general discussion by group.
   3. Review of new habits established and habits still to be established by participants.
   4. Repeat assignment of executing a "right-brain" activity as described in Session 7.
   5. Benediction.
   NOTE: All participants to be given VCE in this interval between 10th and 11th session.

Session 11

   1. The powerful phenomenon of love

VCE Score = 400–150
    a. Words of love almost never used and when rarely used, sound wooden, although quite able to speak even baby talk in affectionate terms to pets.
    b. "I show my love by what I do for him or her."
    c. Physical affection difficult unless sexual.
    d. Voicing criticism, when thought necessary, is much easier to do than expressing affection or even appreciation.

VCE Score = 149–100
    a. Beginning awareness that rewards of any kind do not substitute for physically or vocally expressed love and affection.
    b. Beginning change in belief that expressing love may "spoil" a family member. Shows love even before he or she deserves it.
    c. Less embarrassment in saying in a straightforward fashion, "I love you."

VCE Score = 99–0
    a. Growing belief that expressions of love and affection are the wellsprings of life.
    b. Easy substitution of free-floating affection for prior free-floating hostility.
    c. Now, without embarrassment, can tell spouse, one's child, or even a friend of one's own sex, "I love you."
    d. Recognizes that her/his previous hostility or sense of competition made saying "I love you" difficult.

2. Group inspection of the VCE of each participant: The group and the group counselor will observe and point out every remaining manifestation of TAB in each participant to emphasize what needs additional effort in each participant.

3. Benediction.

Session 12

1. Finish VCE inspections and discussions of each participant.
2. Farewell message of group counselor:
    a. Encourage continuation of doing exercises to rid oneself of old bad habits.
    b. The monitor is the lasting heritage of the total course.
    c. Encourage the principle of transcendence beyond oneself.
3. Benediction.

Appendix 1

Exercises for Modification of Time Urgency and Free-Floating Hostility and Enhancement of Security/Self-Esteem

FOR MODIFICATION OF TIME URGENCY

1. Leave watch off.
2. Walk more slowly.
3. Eat more slowly.
4. Practice having a relaxed face—check in the mirror.
5. Speak more slowly and employ a pleasant tone in your voice. Tape record yourself reading newspaper or book paragraph, then listen to it.
6. Discontinue fist clenching/knee jiggling.
7. Seek a long line (store, bank). On the wall of the Library of Congress is engraved, "If you can't stand being alone, maybe you bore other people, too."
8. Linger at the table.
9. Identify and study the most relaxed person at work or in a social situation.
10. Listen to music and do nothing else for 15 minutes.
11. Think of any past failure and determine whether impatience or hostility played a part.
12. Listen to every person, including spouse and children, without interrupting them.

13. Listen to everyone, including spouse and children, without finishing their sentences.

14. Ask to accompany your spouse to supermarket or substitute for her going.

NOTE: Exercise 14 to be added to the exercises for the second year.

FOR MODIFICATION OF FREE-FLOATING HOSTILITY

1. Ask member of family about their day's activities. If there are family members who are students, look up one of their subjects in your encyclopedia.

2. Verbalize affection to spouse/children.

3. Purposely say, "Maybe I'm wrong," several times in your conversations.

4. Verbalize affection to spouse/partner/children.

5. Note carefully persons, pets, and plants.

6. Find and cultivate a friend (of your own sex) with whom you can share all your confidences and problems.

7. Write a letter to a friend or relative.

8. Observe various people during the day for signs of TAB.

9. Compliment at least two persons.

10. Do something today that is so different from your usual habits that it surprises your family.

11. Substitute compassion and understanding for anger.

12. Ask your spouse what you can do to make his or her life more enjoyable. DON'T ARGUE WITH RESPONSES.

13. Ask opinions of spouse and children about a problem even though you already know the solution. Don't argue, compliment them.

14. List all the faults and also the virtues of your spouse or partner and then destroy the list.

15. Ask spouse or partner if there is anything you can do to make his or her life more pleasant.

16. Just before you are about to criticize a person, avoid doing so.

NOTE: Exercises 13–16 to be added to the exercises for the second year.

FOR ENHANCEMENT OF
SECURITY/SELF-ESTEEM

1. Alter one of your usual habits or ways of doing things.

2. Practice smiling as you remember two to three happy events of the past. Always recall the same happy events.

3. Compliment yourself for some past event or trait before leaving home in the morning.

4. Contemplate your positive achievements for 10 minutes.

5. Recall memories of high school and college for 10 minutes.

6. Set aside 30 minutes for yourself.

7. Read at least two chapters of a book.

8. Enumerate all your qualities that you think are admirable.

9. Begin reading one of these books:
   - Emerson's essays
   - Montaigne's essays
   - Any novel of Dickens, George Eliot, Joan Didion, or Updike John

10. Write out the negative aspects of your life. Bring them to next class for discussion.

11. Catalogue all the good and positive things in your life.

12. Relate to your spouse, children, or a good friend one or more of your past successes or achievements.

13. Ask yourself with whom you really would like to exchange your respective life situations. List reasons for your reluctance.

14. Re-see your house/apartment, its contents, and so on, as if you were a guest. Note the interesting, beautiful, or joyful items.

15. Purposely do or accomplish something that you think may make a pleasant memory.

NOTE: Exercises 9–15 to be added to the exercises for the second year.

Appendix 2

Sample of One Week's Exercises (Drills) to Be Performed

JANUARY (first year)

Monday: Alter one of your usual habits or ways of doing things.

Tuesday: Ask member of family about their day's activities.

Wednesday: Leave watch off.

Thursday: Walk more slowly.

Friday: Verbalize affection to spouse/children.

Saturday: Eat more slowly.

Sunday: Practice smiling as you remember two to three happy events of the past.

General Truths and Principles of Conduct

1. "For every minute you are angry, you lost 60 seconds of happiness."—Ralph W. Emerson
2. "Contempt for others is a weed that can flourish in only one very special kind of soil, that composed of self-contempt."
3. "One can stroke persons with words."—F. Scott Fitzgerald
4. "When a fixed idea makes its appearance, a great ass also makes its appearance."—Nietzsche

Appendix 3

Suggestions and Explanation Concerning Various Exercises

FOR MODIFICATION OF TIME URGENCY

Exercise 5. Once a type A participant who speaks too rapidly (i.e., speaks more than 140 words per minute) listens to his rapid speech on tape (particularly if the tape also records a more normally paced speaker), he recognizes that he actually does speak too quickly. If the counselor observes that a type A group participant continues to speak too rapidly, he should advise the participant to listen repeatedly to his taped speech.

Exercise 7. To type A participants afflicted with time urgency, execution of this exercise at first glance appears totally stupid. This is because he believes he is needlessly wasting time. But when the Congressional aphorism is cited, he has to face up to the fact that he actually does find it boring to be with himself. He must be instructed that the time required for waiting in a line offers a splendid opportunity for him to recall various pleasant episodes in his past or to observe the faces and actions of other waiting persons. The impatient type A repeatedly destroys his past in favor of concerning himself with future contingencies.

FOR MODIFICATION OF FREE-FLOATING HOSTILITY

Exercise 3. The type A participant whose hostility component is severe abhors admitting he is in error. This is due to his underlying inadequate self-esteem. Getting the participant to declare he is wrong, even when he may not be, makes it far easier for him, when he is wrong, to easily admit his error.

Exercise 4. It is often difficult for a type A participant to tell his spouse at luncheon or dinner how deeply he loves her or how much she has gladdened his life. This marital "shyness" requires the frequent conscious execution of this exercise before it becomes a natural mode of giving and receiving affection.

Exercise 5. We have found it efficacious to introduce this exercise by stating that if individuals cease observing these three "Ps," they essentially will not differ from rocks.

Exercise 9. Often type A persons are so prone to criticize that they lose the facility of praising other persons. Hence, they rarely receive compliments themselves, which further diminishes their self-esteem.

FOR ENHANCEMENT OF SECURITY/SELF-ESTEEM

Exercise 7. Except in rare situations, the acquisition of wisdom is not achieved by casual conversations with fellow business or professional acquaintances. It is achieved by the reading of books, selected radio and television programs, and attendance at certain plays and lectures. Often time-urgent type A participants neglect these reservoirs of information. Often their impatience has been so predominant that the reading of a classic becomes almost impossible.

Exercise 13. Few type A persons are willing to exchange their life situations with those of any of their acquaintances. This self-realization helps to enhance their self-esteem.

Appendix 4

General Truths and Principles of Conduct

1. "For every minute you are angry, you lose 60 seconds of happiness." — Ralph W. Emerson

2. "Contempt for others is a weed that can flourish in only one very special kind of soil, that composed of self-contempt."

3. "One can stroke persons with words." — F. Scott Fitzgerald

4. "When a fixed idea makes its appearance, a great ass also makes its appearance." — Nietzsche

5. "There are two species in nature that exhibit impatience, man and puppies. But even a spring bud knows restraint in a prolonged cold spell."

6. "A mind without memories means a body without sensibility." — Herbert Read

7. "No psychic value can disappear without being replaced by another of equal intensity." — C. Jung

8. "The moment numeration ceases to be your servant, it becomes your tyrant."

9. "Love is nature's second sun causing a spring of virtues where he shines." — G. Chapman

10. "An obsession only too often parades as a virtue."

11. "The stature of a man can be measured by the size of an event that preoccupies him."

12. "Good conversation should be a dialogue, not a combat of monologues."

13. "Take joy for just one completed project and do not diminish it by your anxiety of projects still to be completed."

14. "As for disputatious persons, they get victory sometimes, but they never get good will, which would be more use to them."—Ben Franklin

15. "In persons of quality, substance and form cannot be separated."—H. Kissinger

16. "There is no learning to live without learning to love."—J. Powell, SJ

17. "Common sense is wisdom applied to conduct."

18. "One's personal identity is a chain of particular memories."—J. Locke

19. "The creative act is one of liberation—the defeat of habit by originality."—A. Koestler

20. "No one ever learns while talking."

21. "Perhaps the best test of man's intelligence is his capacity for making a summary."—L. Strachey

22. "Ask yourself why you are so much more aware of the irritating qualities than the good qualities of other persons."

23. "The time to examine your belief system is immediately after you have received an unpleasant emotional reaction to some event."

24. "Imagination is more important than knowledge."—A. Einstein

25. "No family can endure if it is bound together by ties of dutiful lovelessness."

26. "The causes of a neurosis lie in the present as well as in the past and only still existing causes can keep a neurosis alive." —C. Jung

27. "Willpower consists of issuing willful, often unpleasant commands and directions to oneself."

28. "Generals would do well to remember that even in war, wisdom comes by opportunity of leisure."—Field Marshal Slim

29. "Beware of the mind-destroying drug of constant activity."—Loren Eisley

30. "Enthusiasm is a passionate eagerness proceeding from an intense conviction of the worthiness of a project. Unlike impatience, it is without irritability or irascibility."

31. "What man betrays or discards his own dog for a younger, more attractive or cleverer dog?"

32. "The greatest of faults is to be conscious of none."

33. "Confronted by outstanding merit in another, there is no way of saving one's ego except by love."—J. Goethe

34. "The power to be truly free is often directly related to the number of human beings you are dependent upon."

35. "To be only for oneself is to be almost nothing."—B. F. Skinner

36. "He who would live in peace and ease must not speak all he knows nor judge all he sees."—Ben Franklin

37. "I cannot trust a man to control others who cannot control himself."—Robert E. Lee

38. "The wicked are always surprised to find that the good can be clever."

39. "Experience, to me, is everyone I meet, if it contains a kernel."—Emily Dickinson

40. "Wisdom always embraces, as one of its *indispensable* components, the processes of pity and forgiveness."

41. "The more flexible and open a person is, the more insights he will acquire."—J. Powell, SJ

42. "The most difficult thing in life is to know yourself."—Thales

43. "Whoever is in a hurry shows that the thing he is about is too big for him."—Lord Chesterfield

44. "True friendship is a plant of slow growth."—George Washington

45. "He who is hurried cannot walk gracefully."—Chinese proverb

46. "A man, who can remember what he has seen, can never be lonely or be without food for thought."—Van Gogh

47. "No new truth is ever really learned until it is acted upon."—J. Powell, SJ

48. "Such good things can happen to people who learn to remember."—Emily Dickinson

49. "And when all the clocks and calendars have stopped their counting for you, what then has your life counted up to?"

50. "God gave us memory so that we can have flowers in the December."—Percy B. Shelley

51. "A life that is not self-examined, self-criticized is not a life worth living."—Plato

52. Imagine a film showing the last ten years of your life. Would you like to see it?"

53. "We can have as many selves as we value other totally different persons."

54. "At the end we shall have enough of cynicism, skepticism and humbug and want life to be more like music."—Van Gogh

55. "God's greatest gift to me is the ability to be astonished anew by the almost incredible beauty of a dandelion plant in full bloom."—Charles Burchfield

56. "Could, by any chance, culture be the meaning and purpose of the second half of our life?"—C. Jung

57. "There is, in my view, one thing you can depend on: people who are interested in power are not interested in people."—J. Ward

58. "We may be in the Universe, as our dogs and cats are in our libraries, seeing the books and hearing the conversation but having no inkling of the meaning of it all."—W. James

59. "You are probably wasting your time if you read any book that you couldn't bear to re-read."

60. "Nothing is so vulgar as to be in a hurry."—Oliver Wendell Holmes

61. "There is a great difficulty for a person to have a purpose in his future if he has no sense of accomplishment in his past."

62. "It is only with the heart that one can see rightly. What is essential is invisible to the eye."—Saint Exupery

63. "When men have killed joy, I do not believe they still live."—Sophocles

64. "Habit is the hardiest of all the plants in human growth."—M. Proust

65. "There are so many *around* us in our life but so very few persons *in* our life."

66. "A person's ambition is only monstrous if it extends hopelessly beyond the paradigm of the possible."

67. "If our measurements and documentations do manage to do away with all our religious beliefs, just what have we gained?"

68. "The most devastating loneliness comes when one never allows himself to be alone."

69. "He who insists on accuracy of trivia, or correction of minute errors in speech, destroys the soul of social communion."

70. "There is no second act in American lives."—F. Scott Fitzgerald

71. "The religion of the rich is the freedom from dread."—Norman Mailer

72. "The most exquisite folly is wisdom spun too finely."—Ben Franklin

73. "My principle is: For heaven's sake, do not be perfect but by all means try to be complete, whatever that means."—C. Jung

74. "To be completely honest with oneself is the very best effort a human being can make."—Sigmund Freud

75. "Think of persons as adventures."—L. Durrell

76. "When a man cannot distinguish a great from a small event, he is of no use to me."—Winston Churchill

77. "The only love that counts for anything is that which reveals itself not just in deed but also in words."

78. "Friendship in the middle class mind is inseparable from respect."—M. Proust

79. "Every good habit that is worth possessing must be paid for in strokes of daily effort."—Charles Darwin

80. "The greatest discovery of our generation is that human beings, by changing the inner attitudes of their minds, can change their lives."

81. "A man never rids himself of hate by eliminating his object of hate."

82. "Very few of the things worth measuring can be measured or even counted."

83. "To thine ownself be true and it must follow as the night the day, thou canst not be false to any man."—William Shakespeare

84. "Knowledge is folly except Grace guide it."—G. Herbert

85. "The only future we can conceive is built upon the forward shadow of our past."—M. Proust

86. "If you make the organization your life, you are defenseless against the inevitable disappointments."—Peter Drucker

87. "Construct standards for other people that are lower than your own."

88. "To go through life viewing yourself as slightly ridiculous is probably one of the best ways to avoid tragedies."

89. "Although the change of qualities to quantities has been proceeding for over three centuries, one can never change back quantities to qualities."

90. "When the Hindus build a temple, they leave one corner unfinished; only God makes something perfect."—C. Jung

91. "We often should be able to say, 'I used to think that but now I think differently.'"

92. "Our children allow us to feel our blood, our friends permit us to glimpse at our soul."

93. "If you are ashamed to pray for something, it may not be worth obtaining."

94. "The test of a first rate mind is to hold two opposing ideas and still be at peace."—F. Scott Fitzgerald

95. "Practice the *form* to achieve the *essence* of tranquility."

96. "Striving for quality never leads to the frenzy arising from striving for quantity."

Appendix 5

The Bait and Hook

1. *Bait Situation*: Anger and criticism from others.
   Examples: Spouse irritated at type A's long hours at work; colleague criticizes work performance.
   Type A Hook Attitude: Hurt and angered by the lack of understanding of his spouse and his colleagues.
2. *Bait Situation*: Messiness or disorder.
   Examples: Spouse fails to sufficiently organize household; children leave toys, games, etc., in disorderly manner.
   Type A Hook Attitude: Upset and intolerant of what he considers lack of organization and order in his home.
3. *Bait Situation*: Others making trivial mistakes.
   Examples: Spouse forgets to pick up shirts from laundry. Colleague makes insignificant error in the office.
   Type A Hook Attitude: Becomes hypercritical and irritated by the failure of spouse's and subordinates' trivial errors of omission or commission.
4. *Bait Situation*: Ideology (political, religious, etc.)
   Examples: Friends express different political views. Type A person reads article describing the religious or cultural beliefs of a different group.
   Type A Hook Attitude: Becomes irascibly intolerant of other people's views and beliefs that differ from his own.
5. *Bait Situation*: Being pressed for time or under a deadline.
   Examples: Project deadline at work; struggling to arrive for an appointment on time.
   Type A Hook Attitude: Becomes at first impatient and then becomes truly angry/hostile to any impediment delaying the pace of his actions.

6. *Bait Situation*: The perceived or comparative slowness of others.
   Examples: Store clerks who move at a slower or calm pace; drivers who drive at the posted speed limit.
   Type A Hook Attitude: The slowness of such persons appears unreasonable and inconsiderate and hence provokes irritation and anger/hostility.
7. *Bait Situation*: The inconsiderate acts of others.
   Examples: People littering; drivers parking in such a way as to occupy too much space.
   Type A Hook Attitude: Becomes angry/hostile at what he believes are inconsiderate acts of these persons.
8. *BaitSituation*: Attempted or perceived manipulation by others.
   Examples: A salesman attempting to push for a sale; spouse tries to persuade type A person to agree with her.
   Type A Hook Attitude: Feels pushed by their attempts to persuade him to do what they wish, hence becomes resentful.

References

Ahern, D. K., Gorkin, L., Anderson, J. L., Tieny, C., Hallstrom, A., Ewart, C., Capone, R. J., Schron, E., Kornfeld, D., Herd, A., Richardson, D. W., & Follick, M. J. (1990). Behavioral variants and mortality in the cardiac arrhythmia pilot study (CAPS). *American Journal of Cardiology*, **66**, 59–67.

Barefoot, J. C., Dahlstrom, W. G. & Williams, R. B. (1983). Hostility, CHD incidence and total mortality: A 25-year follow-up study of 255 physicians. *Psychosomatic Medicine*, **45**, 59–63.

Barefoot, J. C., Peterson, B. L., Harrell, F. E., Hlatky, M. A., Pryor, D. B., Haney, T. L., Blumenthal, J. C., Siegler, I. C., Williams, R. B. (1989). Type A behavior and survival. A follow-up study of 1,467 patients with coronary artery disease. *American Journal of Cardiology*, **64**, 559–570.

Blumenthal, J. A., Williams, R. B., Kong, L., Shanberg, S. W., and Thompson, L. W. (1978). Type A behavior pattern and coronary atherosclerosis. *Circulation*, **58**, 634–639.

Cannon, W. (1915). *Bodily changes in pain, hunger, fear and rage*. New York: Appleton.

Case, R. B., Heller, S. S., Case, N. B. and Moss, A. J. (1985). Type A behavior and survival after acute myocardial infarction. *New England Journal of Medicine*, **313**, 737–741.

Chesney, M., Black, G., Frautschi, N., & De Busk, R. (1986). *Type A and type B women*. Report read at Society of Behavioral Medicine, Washington, DC.

Darwin, F. (Ed.). (1903). *More letters of Charles Darwin*. London: John Murray.

Dembroski, T. M., MacDougall, J. M., Costa, P. T., & Grandits, G. A. (1989). Components of hostility as predictors of sudden death and myocardial infarction in the multiple risk factor intervention trial. *Psychosomatic Medicine*, **51**, 514–522.

Dickinson, E. (1970). *The complete poems of Emily Dickenson*. London: Faber & Faber.

Dreyfuss, F., & Czazkes, J. W. (1959). Blood cholesterol and uric acid on healthy medical students under the stress of an examination. *Archives of Internal Medicine*, **103**, 708–711.

Eaker, E. D., & Castelli, W. P. (1988). Type A behavior and coronary heart disease in women: Fourteen-year incidence from the Framingham study. In B. K. Houston & C. R. Snyder (Eds.), *Type A behavior pattern: Research theory and intervention* (pp. 83–97) New York: John Wiley & Sons.

Eisely, L. (1969). Activism and the rejection of history. *Science*, **165**, 130.

Eliot, G. (1982). *Middlemarch*. New York: Bantam Classics.

Emerson, R. W. (1981). *The portable Emerson*. New York: Penguin Books.

Enos, W. F., Beyer, J. C., & Holmes, R. H. (1955). Pathogenesis of coronary disease in American soldiers killed in Korea. *Journal of the American Medical Association*, **158**, 912–914.

Feinstein, A. R. (1988). Scientific standards in epidemiological studies of the menace of daily life. *Science*, **242**, 1257–1263.

Frank, K., Heller, S., Kornfeld, D., Sporn, A., & Weiss, M. (1976). Type A behavior pattern and coronary angiographic findings. *Journal of the American Medical Association*, **240**, 761–763.

Friedman, M., Byers, S. O., & Rosenman, R. H. (1965). Effects of unsaturated fats upon lipemia and conjunctival circulation. *Journal of the American Medical Association*, **193**, 882–886.

Friedman, M., Byers, S. O., & Rosenman, R. H. (1972). Plasma ACTH and cortisol concentration of coronary-prone subjects. *Proceedings of the Society for Experimental Biology and Medicine*, **140**, 681–684.

Friedman, M., & Ghandour, G. (1993). The medical diagnosis of type A behavior. *American Heart Journal*, **126**, 607–618.

Friedman, M., & Rosenman, R. H. (1959). Association of specific overt behavior pattern with blood and cardiovascular findings. *Journal of the American Medical Association*, **169**, 1286–1296.

Friedman, M., & Rosenman, R. H. (1974). *Type A behavior and your heart*. New York: Knopf.

Friedman, M., Rosenman, R. H., & Byers, S. O. (1964). Serum lipids and conjunctival circulation after fat ingestion in men exhibiting type A behavior pattern. *Circulation*, **29**, 874–866.

Friedman, M., Rosenman, R. H., & Carroll, V. (1958). Changes in the serum cholesterol and blood-clotting time in men subjected to cyclic variation of occupational stress. *Circulation*, **17**, 852–861.

Friedman, M., St. George, S., Byers, S. O., & Rosenman, R. H. (1960). Excretion of catecholamines, 17 ketosteroids, 17 hydroxy-corticoids and 5 hydroxy-indole in men exhibiting a particular behavior pattern (A) associated with high incidence of clinical coronary heart disease. *Journal of Clinical Investigation*, **39**, 758–764.

Friedman, M., Thoresen, C. E., Gill, J. J., Ulmer, D., Powell, L. H., Price, V. A., Brown, B., Thomason, L., Rabin, D. B., Breall, W. S., Bourg, E., Levy, R., & Dixon, J. (1986). Alteration of type A behavior and its effect on cardiac recurrences in postmyocardial infarction patients. Summary results of the Recurrent Coronary Prevention Project. *American Heart Journal*, **112**, 653–665.

Friedman, M., & Ulmer, D. (1984). *Treating type A behavior and your heart*. New York: Knopf.

Fukudo, S., Lane, J. D., Anderson, N. B., Kuhn, C. M., Suzuki, J., & Williams, R. B. (1992). Antagonism of β-adrenergic effect on ventricular repolarization. *Circulation*, **85**, 2045–2053.

Gatson, J. W., & Teevan, R. E. (1980). Type A coronary-prone behavior and fear-of-failure. *Motivation and Emotions*, **4**, 71–76.

Gill, J. J., Price, V. A., Friedman, M., Thoresen, C. E., Powell, L. H., Ulmer, D., Brown, B., & Drews, F. R. (1985). Reduction in type A behavior in healthy, middle-aged American military officers. *American Heart Journal*, **110**, 503–514.

Grundy, S. M., & Griffin, A. C. (1959). Effect of periodic mental stress on serum cholesterol levels. *Circulation* **19**, 496–498.

Grundy, S. M., & Griffin, A. C. (1959b). Relationship of periodic mental stress to serum lipoprotein and cholesterol levels. *Journal of the American Medical Association*, **171**, 1794–1796.

Haynes, S. G., Feinleib, M., Levine, S., Scotch, N., & Kannel, W. B. (1980). The relationship of psychosocial factors to coronary heart disease in the Framingham study. III. Eight year incidence of coronary heart disease. *American Journal of Epidemiology*, **111**, 37–58.

Hearn, M. D., Murray, D. M., & Luepker, R. V. (1989). Hostility, coronary heart disease and total mortality: A 33-year follow-up study of university students. *Journal of Behavioral Medicine*, **12**, 105–121.

Heberden, W. (1772). Some account of a disorder of the breast. In *Medical Transactions* (pp. 59–67). London: College of Physicians.

Helmer, D. C., Ragland, D. H., & Syme, L. L. (1991). Hostility and coronary artery disease. *American Journal of Epidemiology*, **133**, 112–122.

Houston, B. K., & Kelly, K. E. (1987). Type A behavior in housewives: Relation to work, marital adjustment, stress, tension, health, fear of failure and self-esteem. *Journal of Psychosomatic Research*, **31**, 35–61.

Houston, B. K., & Vavack, C. R. (1991). Cynical hostility: Developmental factors, psychosocial correlates, and health behaviors. *Health Psychology*, **10(1)**, 9–17.

James, W. (1890). *The principle's of psychology*. New York: Holt.

Jung, C. G. (1918). *Memories, dreams, reflections*. New York: Vantage Press.

Kaplan, B. (1992). Social health and the forgiving heart: The type B story. *Journal of Behavioral Medicine*, **15**, 3–14.

Kearns, D. (1976). *Lyndon Johnson and the American dream*. New York: Harper & Row.

Knisely, M. H., Bloc, E. H., Eliot, T. S., & Warner, T. (1947). Sludged blood. *Science*, **106**, 431–435.

Leon, G. P., Finn, S. E., Murray, I., & Bailey, J. M. (1988). The inability to predict cardiovascular disease from hostility scores of MMPI items related to type A behavior. *Journal of Consulting Clinical Psychology*, **56**, 567–600.

MacKenzie, J. (1923). *Angina pectoris*. London: Froude, Hodder & Stoughton.

McCramie, E. W., Watkins, L., Brandsma, J., & Sisson, B. (1986). Hostility, coronary heart disease (CHD) incidence and total mortality: Lack of association in a 25-year follow-up study of 478 physicians. *Journal of Behavioral Medicine*, **9**, 119–125.

McNeel, B. J., Keller, B., & Adelstein, S. J. (1975). Primer on certain elements of medical decision making. *New England Journal of Medicine*, **297**, 211–215.

Montaigne, M. (1958). *Essays*. New York: Penguin Books.

Moss, G. E., Dielman, T. E., Campanelli, P. C., Leech, S. L., Harian, W. R., Van Harrison, R., & Horvath, W. J. (1986). Demographic correlates of SI assessments of type A behavior. *Psychosomatic Medicine*, **48**, 564–574.

Osler, W. (1897). *Lectures on angina pectoris*. New York: Appleton.

Popper, K. (1961). *The poverty of historicism*. London: Rutledge & Kegan Paul.

Powell, L. H., Shaker, L. A., Jones, B. A., Vaccarino, L. V., Thoresen, C. E., & Pattillo, J. R. (1993). Psychosocial indicators of mortality in 83 women with premature acute myocardial infarction. *Psychosomatic Medicine*, **55**, 426–433.

Price, V. A. (1982). *Type A behavior pattern: A model for research and practice*. New York: Academic Press.

Price, V. A., Friedman, M., Fleischmann, N., & Ghandour, G. (1995). The relationship between insecurity and type A behavior. *American Heart Journal*, **129**, 488–491.

The Review Panel on Coronary-Prone Behavior and Coronary Heart Disease. (1981). Coronary-prone behavior and coronary heart disease: A critical review. *Circulation*, **63(6)**, 1199–1215.

Rosenman, R. H., Brand, R. J., Jenkins, C. D., Friedman, M., Straus, R., & Wurm, M. (1975). Coronary heart disease in the Western Collaborative Group Study. *Journal of the American Medical Association*, **233**, 872–877.

Ruberman, W., Weinblatt, E., Goldberg, J. D., & Chandhary, B. S. (1984). Psychosocial influences on mortality after myocardial infarction. *New England Journal of Medicine*, **311**, 552–559.

Scherwitz, L. (1986). Interview stylistics and type A predictiveness for CHD incidence clues for an engagement hypothesis. Presented to Kansas Series in Clinical Psychology, Lawrence, Kansas, May 10–11.

Shekelle, R., Hully, S. B., Neaton, J. D., Billings, J. H., Borhani, N. D., Gerace, T. A., Jacobs, D. R., Lasher, N. L., Mittlemark, M. B., & Stamler, J. (1985). The MRFIT behavior pattern study. II. Type A behavior and incidences of coronary heart disease. *American Journal of Epidemiology*, **122**, 559–570.

Smith, G. D., Phillips, A. N., & Neaton, J. D. (1992). Smoking as "independent" risk factor for suicide. Illustration of an artifact from observational epidemiology. *Lancet*, **1**, 709–712.

Swets, L. A., & Pichett, R. M. (1982). *Evaluation of diagnostic systems: Methods from signal detection theory*. New York: Academic Press.

Thoresen, C. E., & Low, K. G. (1990). Type A behavior. *Journal of Social Behavior and Personality*, **5**(1), 117–133.

Twain, M. (1982). *Life on the Mississippi*. New York: The Library of America.

Westlake, P. T., Wilcox, A. A., Haley, M. I., & Peterson, J. E. (1958). Relationship of mental and emotional stress to serum cholesterol levels. *Proceedings of Society of Experimental Biology and Medicine*, **97**, 163–165.

Williams, R. B., Haney, T. L., & Lee, K. L. (1988). Type A behavior, hostility and coronary atherosclerosis. *Psychosomatic Medicine*, **42**, 539–549.

Williams, R. B., Lane, J. D., Kuhn, C. M., Meosh, W., White, A. D., & Schamberg, S. N. (1982). Type A behavior and elevated physiological and neuroendocrine responses to cognitive tasks. *Science*, **218**, 483–486.

Zumoff, B., Rosenfeld, R. N., Friedman, M., Byers, S. O., Rosenman, R. H., & Hellman, L. (1984). Elevated daytime urinary excretion of testosterone gluconide in men with type A behavior pattern. *Psychosomatic Medicine*, **40**, 223–225.

Index

Accountants, cholesterol levels in, 7
Acetylcholine, 5
Achievement
   as insecurity response, 25–26, 29
   memories of, 16, 36, 46, 62–63
   of others, 29
   as parental affection substitute,
     21–22
ACTH (adrenocorticotrophic hormone),
   5–6, 12
Activities
   of human mind, 108–109
   prioritization of, 71, 103, 107, 109
   temporal importance of, 72
Addison's disease, 5–6
Admiration
   parental
     toward type B behavior individuals,
       13–14
     type A behavior individuals' lack of,
       20–22, 61–62
   type A behavior individuals' inability to
     express, 28, 29, 80
Adrenocorticotrophic hormone (ACTH),
   5–6, 12
Affection, 13–14
   expressed by group counseling leaders,
     56
   from others, 46, 86
   parental
     toward type B behavior individuals,
       13–14
     type A behavior individuals' lack of,
       20–22, 46, 59–62

Affection (*cont.*)
   toward friends, 63–64, 109, 122–123
   toward pets, 86, 109
   toward spouse, 64, 80, 132
   type A behavior individuals' inability to
     express, 28, 29, 80, 132
   verbalization of, 109
AIAI (anger, irritability, aggravation, im-
     patience) mnemonic, of type
     A behavior, 71, 97–98, 106,
     110
Altruism, disbelief in, 30, 41
Anger
   justified, 79, 84
   type A behavior individuals' attitudes
     toward, 139
   See also Hostility, free-floating
Anger-inducing incidents, intensity of re-
     action to, 79
Angina, 9, 11, 19
Anxiety, 23
Apprehension: *see* Proleptic behavior
Army officers, type A behavior
     counseling intervention study of,
     92–94
Atherosclerosis
   erythrocyte agglutination in, 10–11
   in women, 19

Belief systems, substitution of new for
     old, 98, 102, 106
   for free-floating hostility modification,
     79–81
   for self-esteem enhancement, 61–64

145

Group counseling, for type A behavior
modification (*cont.*)
for Army officers, 92–96 (*cont.*)
relaxation techniques in, 101, 102,
105, 106, 107, 108, 110
second year, 109–124
use of Videotaped Clinical Examination in, 97, 102, 110–113, 115–124
Group leaders
at Friedman Institute, 58
qualities of, 55–58
role in driving-related time urgency
modification, 74–75
role in self-monitor construction,
65
use of philosophical quotations and
maxims by, 66–67
Growth hormone, 6–7

Habit-forming exercises
for free-floating hostility modification,
82–83
for self-esteem enhancement, 65–66
for time urgency modification, 73,
125–126
Hormones
in type A behavior, 4–6
in type B behavior, 12
Hostility, free-floating, 4, 23, 27–30
behavioral manifestations of, 78
in children, 21, 59
as coronary heart disease risk factor,
25, 32–33
diagnosis of, 33-35, 40–44
elicitation of symptoms and traits,
40–41
of psychomotor signs, 42–44
during driving, 29
modification of, 73–75, 99–100, 101
facial expressions of, 42, 43, 44
family relationships and, 27–29, 30
modification of, 65–66, 77–84, 126,
131–132
during driving, 73–75, 99–100, 101
new habit-forming exercises for,
82–83
in social interactions, 112–113
through long-term group counseling,
95, 96

Hostility, free-floating (*cont.*)
modification of, 65–66, 77–84, 126,
131–132 (*cont.*)
through substitution of new for old
belief systems, 79–81
psychomotor signs of, 50–51
diagnosis of, 42–44
modification of, 83, 96
self-recognition of, 78
self-monitoring of, 50, 78, 79, 81–82
type B behavior individuals' lack of, 16, 17
type A behavior group counseling leaders' lack of, 56
Housewives, type A behavior in, 18
Humanities
group counseling leaders' knowledge
of, 57
as right-brain activity, 109
Humor, of type B behavior individuals, 16
Hypercholesterolemia, 6–8
Hypertriglyceridemia, 8–9, 10

Impatience: *see* Time urgency
Inconsiderateness, of others, 140; *see also*
Conduct, breaches of; Mistakes, of
others
Insecurity/inadequate self-esteem, 3,
20–22
achievement as response to, 25–26, 29
diagnosis of, 33, 35, 44–47
in type B behavior individuals, 47
enhancement interventions for, 59–67,
127, 132
contemplation of general truths and
principles of conduct, 66–67
new habit-forming exercises, 65–66
self-monitoring, 59–60, 64–65
substitution of new for old belief systems, 61–64
Videotaped Clinical Examination
scores in, 116–117
relationship to anxiety, 23
relationship to criticism, 22–23
relationship to depression, 23
relationship to time urgency, 25–26
Integrity, of type A behavior group counseling leaders, 56

Type B behavior individuals (*cont.*)
hormonal functions in, 6, 12
psychological characteristics of,
13–18
right-brain activities of, 15–16
triglyceride levels in, 9
free-floating hostility of, 47
personality of, 15
success of, 104
time urgency of, 47

Uncertainty, free-floating hostility as reaction to, 81
United States Army War College, type A
behavior counseling intervention at,
92–94

Videotaped Clinical Examination (VCE),
33–51
for free-floating hostility diagnosis,
33–35, 40–44, 50, 51
for insecurity/inadequate self-esteem diagnosis, 33, 35, 44–47, 50, 51
for time urgency diagnosis, 33–40, 49–50, 51
elicitation of symptoms and traits,
35–36
psychomotor sign evaluation,
36–40
use in Coronary/Cancer Prevention Project, 95, 96
use in Recurrent Coronary Prevention
Project, 89, 90
use in type A behavior group counseling efficacy evaluation
for expression of affection and love,
123
for friendship, 122–123

Videotaped Clinical Examination (VCE)
(*cont.*)
use in type A behavior group counseling efficacy evaluation (*cont.*)
for insecurity/inadequate self- esteem, 116–117
for parenting, 111–112
for personal view of change process, 118
for responses to hooks and unexpected events, 118–119
for social interactions, 112–113
for spirituality, 120–122
for time urgency, 115–116
for vocational success, 119–120
use in U.S. Army War College type A
intervention study, 92, 93, 94
Videotaped structured interview (VSI),
use in Recurrent Coronary Prevention Project, 88
Vocational success
role of type A behavior in, 119–120
of type B behavior individuals, 104
Voice, hostile tone of, 44, 105, 112

Waiting in lines, dislike for, 36
Western religions, 86
Women
erythrocyte agglutination in, 10–11
as type A behavior group counseling
leaders, 58
type A behavior in, 18–19
ability to express affection, 64
free-floating hostility, 51
insecurity/inadequate self-esteem, 51
time urgency, 51, 70–71
Worldview, hostile, modification of, 79–80

Yalow, Rosalyn, 6